Neonatal Pharmacology and Nutrition Update

Pediatric and Adolescent Medicine

Vol. 18

Series Editor

Wieland Kiess Leipzig

Neonatal Pharmacology and Nutrition Update

Volume Editors

Francis B. Mimouni Tel Aviv
Johannes N. van den Anker Washington, DC/Basel/Rotterdam

8 figures, 2 in color, 13 tables, 2015

KARGER Basel · Freiburg · Paris · London · New York · Chennai · New Delhi · Bangkok · Beijing · Shanghai · Tokyo · Kuala Lumpur · Singapore · Sydney

Pediatric and Adolescent Medicine
Founded 1991 by D. Branski, Jerusalem

Francis B. Mimouni
Tel Aviv Medical Center
Dana Dwek Children's Hospital
Tel Aviv, Israel

Johannes N. van den Anker
Children's National Medical Center
Washington, DC, USA
University Children's Hospital
Basel, Switzerland
Erasmus Medical Center – Sophia Children's Hospital
Rotterdam, The Netherlands

Library of Congress Cataloging-in-Publication Data

Neonatal pharmacology and nutrition update / volume editors, Francis B. Mimouni, Johannes N. van den Anker.
p. ; cm. -- (Pediatric and adolescent medicine, ISSN 1017-5989 ; vol. 18)
Includes bibliographical references and indexes.
ISBN 978-3-318-02735-8 (hard cover : alk. paper) -- ISBN 978-3-318-02736-5 (electronic version)
I. Mimouni, Francis, editor. II. Van den Anker, Johannes N., editor. III. Series: Pediatric and adolescent medicine ; v. 18. 1017-5989
[DNLM: 1. Infant, Newborn--metabolism. 2. Pharmacological Phenomena. 3. Infant Formula. 4. Infant, Newborn, Diseases--drug therapy. 5. Pharmaceutical Preparations--administration & dosage. W1 PE163HL v.18 2015 / QV 37]
RJ253
618.92'01--dc23

2014035512

Bibliographic Indices. This publication is listed in bibliographic services, including Current Contents®.

www.karger.com
Printed in Germany on acid-free and non-aging paper (ISO 9706) by Kraft Druck GmbH, Ettlingen
ISSN 1017–5989
e-ISSN 1662–3886
ISBN 978–3–318–02735–8
e-ISBN 978–3–318–02736–5

KARGER 125 YEARS

Contents

Foreword

The authors, editorial board and publisher wish to dedicate this volume in our Pediatric and Adolescent Medicine series, published by Karger Publishers, Basel, Switzerland, to Prof. Dr. David Branski, Jerusalem.

David Branski passed away last year, painfully and much too early, and he is greatly and dearly missed by his family, his friends and his colleagues around the world. David Branski was a professor at Hadassah in Jerusalem, and he was one of the leading pediatric gastroenterologists of our time. He was loved and liked by all who got to know him. His humble and friendly and always-supportive demeanour made him a laudable and highly respected colleague. David inaugurated and supported our Pediatric and Adolescent Medicine book series over many years. I was welcomed by David to join him as a co-editor for our series some years ago. Here, I could witness his warmth, his humble and highly intelligent personality, and his devotion to and liking of children and their families. I also became aware of his deep and wise understanding of science and of scientific medicine.

While we all miss David Branski very much, it was a joy, an honour and very rewarding to have been able to get to know him and to work with him over the years. I am particularly grateful that I was able to welcome David and his wife one summer evening in Leipzig. This, our personal meeting, closed the circle between us and our institutions, the University of Leipzig in Germany and Hadassah Medical Centre in Jerusalem, Israel.

Again, we solemnly dedicate this volume of the Pediatric and Adolescent Medicine series with the title of 'Neonatal Pharmacology and Nutrition Update', edited by Francis B. Mimouni and Johannes N. van den Anker, to the memory of David Branski, to his scientific work and to his collegial friendship.

Wieland Kiess, Leipzig

Preface

In December 2005, on a flight to Brussels, one of us (Francis Mimouni) travelled with Prof. David Branski, of blessed memory, to the board meeting of the European Academy of Pediatrics. David asked Francis if he had any ideas about possible topics for books in the Karger series in Pediatrics. Francis, a neonatologist, immediately felt that one of greatest challenges in Neonatology was the correct use of medications, which for the most part, have never been tested in neonates, and even less so in small, fragile 'micropremies'.

David registered the idea as a 'good one', and in 2011, he contacted Francis. The problem was that Francis was not a real pharmacologist, and his connection with the 'alchemistry' of drugs was through the field of nutrition and metabolism. Francis promptly looked for a partner for this endeavor and found that the specific issues he thought needed to be tackled were the topics of a newly organized course in Pediatric and Neonatal pharmacology at the European Society for Pediatric Research's annual meeting in Newcastle. Well-respected European and US experts gave outstanding lectures during this course, and Francis met Johannes van den Anker, one of only a handful of world-renowned experts in Neonatal Pharmacology. We decided to work together on this book, which is dedicated to Neonatal Pharmacology and Nutrition, and used the program of the ESPR course as a template. To make it even more attractive for the readership, we have added three very relevant chapters to its content: a chapter on the regulation of drug development, another on the rationale and scientific basis for formula development in preterm infants, and a third chapter presenting a systematic review and meta-analysis on the use of paracetamol (acetaminophen) for the medical closure of patent ductus arteriosus.

We hope you will enjoy reading this book, which is dedicated to the memory of our dear friend, Prof. David Branski.

Francis B. Mimouni, Tel Aviv
Johannes N. van den Anker, Washington, DC/Basel/Rotterdam

Mimouni FB, van den Anker JN (eds): Neonatal Pharmacology and Nutrition Update.
Pediatr Adolesc Med. Basel, Karger, 2015, vol 18, pp 1–12 (DOI: 10.1159/000364987)

Influence of Maturation and Growth on Drug Metabolism from Fetal to Neonatal to Adult Life

Synnöve Lindemalm[a] • Johannes N. van den Anker[b–e]

[a]Astrid Lindgren Children's Hospital, Karolinska University Hospital, Stockholm, Sweden; [b]Division of Pediatric Clinical Pharmacology, Children's National Medical Center, Washington, DC, and [c]Departments of Pediatrics, Pharmacology, Physiology and Integrative Systems Biology, George Washington University School of Medicine and Health Sciences, Washington, DC, USA; [d]Intensive Care, Erasmus MC-Sophia Children's Hospital, Rotterdam, The Netherlands; [e]Department of Paediatric Pharmacology, University Children's Hospital, Basel, Switzerland

Abstract

Drug metabolism is the enzymatic conversion of one chemical compound into another, ultimately resulting in a product that can be excreted by the kidneys. In the processes by which the body excretes drugs into fluids such as urine or bile, metabolism is an essential step in converting drugs into more water-soluble compounds by increasing their polarity. This metabolism can be classified into phase I and phase II reactions. The liver is the main organ of interest for metabolism, although some processes occur in the lungs, intestine, kidneys and plasma. For one group of enzymes, the level and activity are greatest during the fetal stage, and for a second group, the activity begins during fetal life, continues after birth and can be observed in adults. For a third group of enzymes, the activity can only be detected after birth, and the highest activity is found in children, adolescents and adults. The unique pattern, ontogeny, and development of the metabolizing enzymes for each substance makes it impossible to generalize data from adults to children. Interindividual variability is immense, particularly among newborns and infants. The maturation of drug-metabolizing enzymes is the most important factor in determining the rate of metabolism and thus in determining the optimum dose for the individual patient.

Clinical Relevance of Ontogeny

In the processes by which the body excretes a drug into fluids such as urine or bile, metabolism is an essential step in converting a drug into a more water-soluble, inactive compound by increasing its polarity, such as in the glucuronidation of chloramphenicol. Metabolism can also result in the transformation of a parent compound or pro-drug into a more active or potent drug, as evidenced by the transformation of codeine into morphine by CYP2D6. However, metabolism can also result in the for-

Table 1. Age classification of patients

Category		Age
Prenatal	first trimester	GA w 0–12
	second trimester	GA w 13–26
	third trimester	GA w 27–40 (partus)
Postnatal	newborn	0–27 days
	infants	28 days–23 months
	children	2–11 years
	adolescents	12–18 years

GA = Gestational age; w = week.

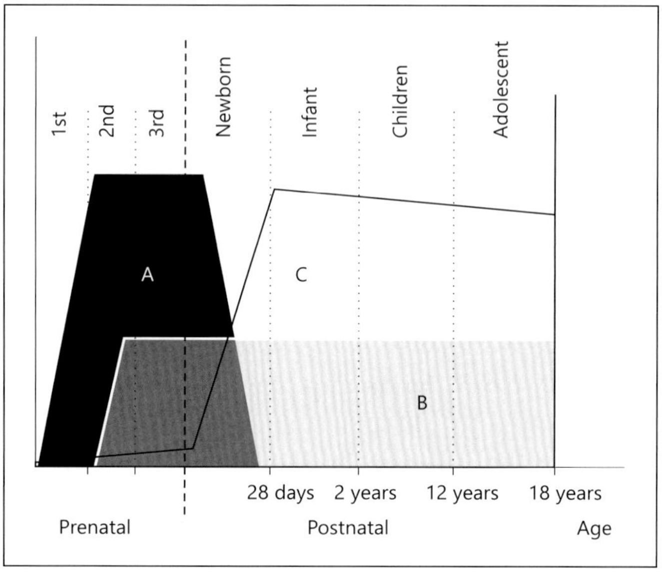

Fig. 1. Category A: Enzymes expressed at high levels during first trimester, remain high during gestation or decrease. Often silent or expressed at low levels within two years postnatally. Category B: Expressed at constant level during gestation age and small changes are observed after birth. Category C: Enzymes expressed at low levels or not at all in the fetus. An increase can be seen for some of the enzymes during second and third trimester, or after birth.

mation of a toxic compound, as in the example of paracetamol hepatotoxicity caused by N-acetyl-p-benzoquinone-imine, which is produced by the action of the oxidative enzyme CYP2E1. This toxic reaction occurs when levels of glutathione are low and/or levels of CYP2E1 are high. The differences between children and adults can often be found in the differences between the ratios of metabolites relative to the parent drug, and in some cases, novel metabolites have been found to be unique to the pediatric population. Age-dependent aspects are therefore of great importance when considering pharmacokinetics, pharmacodynamics or adverse reactions to drug treatment [1–3] (table 1; fig. 1).

Metabolism can be classified into phase I and phase II reactions. Phase I involves the structural change of the molecule through oxidation, reduction or hydrolysis. Cy-

Table 2. Categories of enzymes during maturation and growth

Category		Postnatal age
A	Enzymes expressed at high levels during first trimester, remain high during gestation or decrease. Often silent or expressed at low levels within two years postnatally.	CYP3A7 FMO1 SULT1A3/4 ADH1A
B	Expressed at constant level during gestation age and small changes are observed after birth.	CYP2C19, 3A5 SULT1A1
C	Enzymes expressed at low levels or not at all in the fetus. An increase can be seen for some of the enzymes during second and third trimester, or after birth.	CYP3A, 1A2, 2C9, 2D6, 2E1, 3A4 SULT2A1, 2A1 ADH1C, 1B FMO3

tochrome P450 iso-enzymes are the most important group of enzymes involved in this phase. Esterases and dehydrogenases are other phase I enzymes of importance for metabolism [4]. Phase II reactions consist of conjugation with another, often more water-soluble molecule, as in acetylation, methylation, sulfation or glucuronidation. Uridine diphosphate glucuronosyltransferase (UGT) is one of the major iso-enzymes involved in phase II reactions and is relevant to the metabolism of many drugs such as paracetamol, morphine and chloramphenicol. Furthermore, they are involved in the biotransformation of endogenous compounds such as bilirubin and steroids [5–7].

The liver is the main organ of interest for metabolism, although some processes occur in the lungs, intestine, kidney and plasma.

The expression and activity of drug metabolizing enzymes (DMEs) change significantly during ontogeny, and differences in therapeutic efficacy or adverse drug reactions may occur. To categorize with the aim of simplification, DMEs were divided into one of three groups by Hines [2], as shown in table 2 and figure 1. In the first group, the enzymes are expressed and the highest activity is found in the first trimester, and the enzyme activity remains constant or decreases during gestation. The activity is low or the enzymes are silenced within two years after birth. In the second group, the enzymes are expressed at relatively constant levels throughout gestation, and relatively few changes are observed postnatally. In the third group, the activity is very low or silent during fetal life. The activity and/or expression increase after birth, and a substantial increase in activity is observed within the first years of life.

There are several well-known therapeutic differences in children and in neonates in particular; in these groups, the drug disposition and response can substantially differ from those in adults, with potentially dangerous results. 'Grey baby syndrome', consisting of cyanosis, abdominal distension, abnormal respiration, emesis, cardiovascular collapse and death, is often cited. When safe doses for adults were extrapolated to neonates, the doses were found to be lethal. The primary cause of lethality was found to be the immaturity of the UDP glucuronosyl transferase system, which resulted in impaired drug metabolism and clearance [8]. However, children may also exhibit resistance to toxicity relative to that in adults, as found for acetaminophen due to the capacity for sulfate conjugation early in life [9].

Differences in pharmacokinetic parameters during development contribute substantially to observed changes in efficacy and to adverse drug reactions in children [10].

In this chapter, we will describe some of the enzymes involved in metabolism and present some examples and clinical applications of changes during growth.

Why Metabolism?

General

During fetal life and childhood, the maturation of organ systems has a profound effect on drug disposition. Cytochromes P-450 (CYPs) are mainly responsibility for the biotransformation of hydrophobic molecules, such as endogenous steroids, fatty acids and prostaglandins, and of exogenous chemicals, such as environmental pollutants, carcinogens and drugs [11]. Cytochromes P-450 comprise a group of hemoproteins that mostly catalyze oxidative metabolism. The ontogeny of metabolizing enzymes is most likely the main factor that accounts for non-renal drug clearance [3]. From early fetal life through the first year of life, the total hepatic content of CYP appears to be fairly stable and corresponds to levels between 30 and 60% of those observed in adults [12, 13].

Cytochrome families 1–4 are the most relevant for drug metabolism in humans, and CYP3A4 (52%), CYP2D6 (31%) and CYP2C9 (10%) are the greatest contributors [4, 6].

Challenges with Techniques for Assessing CYP Activity

Different in vitro techniques can be used to assess the impact of development on CYP activity, in which iso-enzyme-specific phenotypic expression of protein, mRNA and protein activity can be evaluated. Hepatic tissues are often collected shortly post-mortem, and the number of samples is often small and covers only a small time window during growth. In vivo examination can also provide valuable information for the evaluation of phenotypic iso-enzyme activity following administration of a probe drug.

Depending on the method used to detect CYP expression, problems with sensitivity or quantitation may occur. Limitations regarding the differentiation of the various CYP isoforms may be present; these may be overcome by the use of specific antibodies [4–6, 10, 14–16].

The ability to simultaneously assess several processes in a controlled setting is a great advantage for the in vitro technique. However, in contrast, the effects of hepatic blood flow or hepatic microstructure on the phenotype are not taken into account. Extrahepatic metabolism, that is, renal, gastrointestinal or pulmonary metabolism, can also contribute to the phenotypic variability, increasing the difficulty of in vivo assessment [4, 6, 10, 14–16].

Table 3. Expression of different CYP enzymes during growth

CYP450	1st	2nd	3rd	Newborn	Infant	Child	Adolescent
2C9	1%	1%	10%	25%	25%	50%	50–100%
2C19	10%	20%	20%	20%	50%	50%	100%
2E1	ND	0–2%	0–10%	25%	100%	100%	100%
3A4	D	D	D	D	D	100%	100%
3A5	0–100%	0–100%	0–100%	0–100%	0–100%	0–100%	100%
3A7	300%*	300%*	200%*	150%*	30%*	30%*	30%*

ND = Not detectable; D = detectable. * Compared to level found for CYP3A4.

CYP3A

The most extensive group of CYP enzymes is CYP3A, which comprises 30–40% of the adult CYP content in the liver and small intestine [17–19]. CYP3A consists of at least three isoforms, CYP3A4, 3A5 and 3A7 [20, 21]. Immunoquantitated fetal CYP3A content, obtained from liver microsomes, ranges from 30 to 100% of that in adults [12, 22].

CYP3A7

CYP3A7 is the major enzyme found in utero and in newborns, but it can also be found in adults, albeit in much lower levels compared to CYP3A4 [23–25]. The nucleotide sequence of CYP3A7 is nearly 90% homologous to that of CYP3A4 [25, 26]. CYP3A7 plays an important role in the biotransformation of endogenous compounds, such as hormones that are important during pregnancy, and it is also capable of metabolizing potential environmental pollutants [27, 28].

CYP3A7 is the dominant enzyme during the prenatal period, with levels of expression that are two to three times higher than those observed for CYP3A4 in adults. In the neonatal and infant periods, CYP3A7 decreases but remains a dominant CYP enzyme. In children, the enzymes shift, and CYP3A4 becomes dominant to CYP3A7, as shown in tables 2, 3 and figure 1 [29].

CYP3A4

CYP3A4 is the most highly expressed CYP in the liver and intestine [19, 30]. The list of substrates metabolized by CYP3A4 is growing rapidly and includes many therapeutically important drugs such as erythromycin, midazolam and cyclosporine, as well as endogenous substrates such as testosterone, cortisol and progesterone [16].

CYP3A4 is mainly found in the upper small intestine as an extrahepatic site, and it is also expressed in the esophagus, duodenum and colon but not in the stomach [17, 18, 31]. The extrahepatic sites of enzyme activity represent up to 40% of the total

CYP3A4 in adults [32]. This could be of clinical importance for bioavailability if the intestinal epithelium is reduced due to diseases such as celiac disease or short bowel syndrome [33].

CYP3A4 can be detected in fetal hepatic tissue in the second or third trimester [33, 34] at approximately 10% of adult levels. CYP3A4 levels rise after birth and reach up to 50% of adult levels within the first year [35–37]. Gestational age does not influence the pattern of activity [35]. In other studies, CYP3A4 was the dominant CYP3 enzyme expressed in children, and adult levels are not achieved until 3 years of age [29].

CYP3A5

CYP3A5 is the main iso-enzyme in the kidney, but it is also found in the lungs, blood, pituitary gland, stomach and esophagus [17, 18, 38, 39]. CYP3A5 is up to 85% similar to CYP3A4, but these enzymes differ substantially in substrate expression and specificity [40]. CYP3A5 can be detected in some samples in the first trimester. In the samples in which the enzyme was expressed, the levels remained intact in both the second and third trimester, and the expression remained intact throughout growth, as shown in tables 2, 3 and in figure 1 [29].

CYP2D6

CYP2D6 represents only 2% of the total hepatic CYP content, but many drugs such as β-blockers, antitussive drugs and tricyclic antidepressants are metabolized by this enzyme that is polymorphically expressed. The protein concentration was immunochemically determined, and the RNA level and the CYP2D6 dependent activity were investigated in a study of 75 liver samples from fetuses aged 17–40 weeks. The concentration of hepatic CYP2D6 protein was low or undetectable in 70% of the tested samples. The protein concentration rose within the first week following birth, and the trend was independent of the gestational age at birth. CYP2D6 RNA was detected earlier than the protein and was found to peak in newborns and to decline in adults [41].

Tramadol hydrochloride (M), an analogue of codeine, can be used as a probe drug in the first months of life to assess CYP2D6 and CYP3A4 ontogeny. Tramadol is metabolized by CYP2D6 to O-demethyl tramadol (M1) and to N-demethyl tramadol (M2), mainly by CYP3A4 [42]. The activity of CYP3A4 is relatively delayed in the first months of life compared to that of CYP2D6 [43, 44].

CYP2E1

CYP2E1 is mainly expressed in the liver but is also found in the lungs [45]; in rats, it is also found in the small intestine and in the brain [31, 46]. Among the drugs metabolized by CYP2E1 are acetaminophen, isoniazid and the halogenated anesthetics halothane and enflurane [47, 48]. CYP2E1 is also involved in the metabolism of aldehydes, alcohols and ketones, and it plays a principal role in gluconeogenesis from endogenous ketone bodies [49].

In 82 liver samples obtained from fetuses, no enzyme activity or CYP2E1 protein could be detected. However, within hours after birth, both protein and enzyme activities were observed [50]. In another study, CYP2E1 expression was not detected in the first trimester but was detected in the second and third trimesters. In neonatal livers, CYP2E1 was increased two to three times and represented 25% of the levels observed in adults. In infants, the levels increased, and in adolescents, the levels matched those observed in adults, as shown in tables 2, 3 and figure 1 [29].

CYP2C9

Many substrates such as phenytoin, ibuprofen and warfarin are metabolized by CYP2C9. Expression of CYP2C9 was low in the first and second trimesters but increased in the third trimester to approximately 10% of the levels found in adults. As for CYP2E1, CYP2C9 increased two to three times in neonates. In young adolescents, the level of CYP2C9 expression was the same as in infants and approximately half that observed in adults, as shown in tables 2, 3 and figure 1 [29].

CYP2C19

Substances such as omeprazole, diazepam and barbiturates are metabolized by CYP2C19. In the first trimester, expression of CYP2C19 was approximately 10% of that found in adults. The level of expression increased slightly in the second trimester to 20% of the levels observed in adults and remained at that level in the third trimester and in newborns. In infants and young adolescents, the expression increased to approximately 50% of the levels in adults, as shown in tables 2, 3 and figure 1 [29].

Oxidative Enzymes Other than Cytochromes P450

Alcohol Dehydrogenase, ADH

The ADH family catalyzes the oxidation and reduction of a wide variety of alcohols and aldehydes. ADH class 1 includes ADHs A-C and is expressed during the prenatal period. During the first trimester, ADH1A was detectable. In the second trimester, all three enzymes were found, but ADH1A was dominant. In the third trimester, the levels of ADH1A and ADH1B were equivalent but greater than those of ADH1C. In adults, the expression of ADH1A was low or was not detectable [51].

Flavin-containing Monooxygenases, FMOs

The family of FMO enzymes is important for the oxidative metabolism of a variety of therapeutics, toxins and endogenous compounds. A developmental transition between FMO1 and FMO3 was first reported fifteen years ago. FMO1 is found predominately in the prenatal period, with the highest activity observed during the first trimester. Birth is important, but is not the only factor, for the onset of FMO3 expression [2].

Phase II Enzymes

Acetylation, glucuronidation, sulfation and methylation are all examples of phase II reactions [5–7, 10].

Uridine 5′-diphospho-glucuronosyltranferases (UGTs) are of great importance for the clearance and elimination of drugs and hormones. In an in vitro study, UGT1A1 enzyme activity was present at birth, although at a very low level, and it increased to a plateau after less than four months. The activity of UGT1A6 was higher at birth but increased to adult levels only after the first year [52]. Despite the differences in activity, there was no relationship between the activity levels and the protein levels.

In almost all newborns, an immature bilirubin UGT combined with an increase in the breakdown of red blood cells manifests in hyperbilirubinemia.

Sulfation is the transfer of a sulfate group from 3′-phosphoadenosine 5′-phosphosulfate to a substrate and is catalyzed by sulfotransferase (SULT) enzymes. Many studies have demonstrated that there is already significant sulfotransferase activity in the second trimester [2]. SULT1A1 is expressed at a relatively constant level during the prenatal period, and a minimal change is observed after birth. The activity of SULT1E1 decreases after birth in contrast to that of SULT2A1, which increases [2].

Glucuronidation of acetaminophen, which is a substrate of UGT1A6 and UGT1A9, and of morphine, which is a substrate of UGT2B7, is lower than that in adults [10, 53].

Paracetamol (acetaminophen), or N-acetyl-p-aminophenol, is the most frequently prescribed drug for the treatment of fever and pain in children [54]. It has many different modes of administration, such as the intravenous, oral and rectal routes, and when metabolized, it is sulfated, glucuronidated or conjugated with glutathione and can therefore provide important information [55–57]. Although paracetamol has been used for more than 100 years, new observations have been made regarding its pharmacodynamics profile. There is evidence that repeated use of paracetamol will result in induction of glucuronidation, and a shift from biliary to urinary elimination of paracetamol glucuronide with repeated administration has been demonstrated in rodents [58, 59].

Highlights during Maturation and Growth

Birth

During the neonatal period, there are rapid physiological changes in liver blood flow, including closure of the ductus venosus. The umbilical blood supply is immediately discontinued after birth, which causes changes in hepatic oxygenation. These changes may cause altered bioavailability in the neonate, but the main impact is most likely on hepatic metabolism. As previously noted, birth itself, either preterm or term, seems to be of great importance for drug metabolism. Postnatal maturation of both CYP and glucuronidation capacity in preterm and term infants illustrates the importance of investigating the impact of both postnatal and postmenstrual age on these developmental changes [60].

The term 'developmental switch' is often used to describe the transition between the enzymes that are dominant during gestation to the enzymes that are dominant after birth. Such a switch is well recognized for CYP3A7, which is highly expressed in the fetus, and CYP3A4, which is the dominant enzyme of the CYP2A family in adults [35]. Similar switches are found for FM01 and FM03 and for CYP2C19 and CYP2C9. This phenomenon is more of a developmental transition because no regulatory mechanism is known to date.

Adolescence

Around the time of puberty, the DMEs gradually begin to decline; this reduction continues throughout adolescence and settles at adult capacity upon the completion of pubertal development. In many studies, hepatically metabolized drugs such as theophylline, carbamazepine, phenytoin and phenobarbital have increased clearance in children (2–11 years of age). Therefore, higher doses are required to achieve the desired effects in children compared to those necessary for adults. However, drug dosing is generally similar to that in young adults by the end of adolescence. Collectively, the data suggest that alterations in DME activity are mediated by sex and/or growth hormones during adolescence [61].

In a Clinical Setting

The ontogeny of DMEs substantially influences pharmacokinetic changes that may contribute to changes in therapeutic efficacy and to adverse drug reactions [2]. Despite several federal initiatives to increase the information about and documentation of drugs administered to children 0–18 years of age, off-label use is common in all groups of children [54]. Gaps remain in the knowledge of the ontogeny of DMEs, and when combined with widespread off-label use and a lack of information, the variability in response to a given treatment is immense. The most vulnerable patients are newborns, children with chronic diseases, and infants, children and adolescents admitted to pediatric intensive care units. It is a challenge for the physician to find the correct dose and give it to the correct patient in the correct manner. If the physician fails to find the correct dose, the patient might suffer for the rest of his/her life from such an error.

The approach to dosing in pediatrics needs to be based on this knowledge, on understanding the effects of ontogeny on DME, on knowledge of the drug and on the characteristics of the child. Every substance is unique and has its own way of being processed by the body, that is, its own pharmacokinetics. The unique pattern of the individual's ontogeny and the development of metabolizing enzymes for each substance make it impossible to generalize data from adults to children. The maturation of enzyme systems is the most important factor in determining the rate of metabolism in neonates and infants, and other factors of importance are hepatic blood flow, hepatic transport systems and hepatic metabolic capacity.

The following are some very simple rules to consider for drugs that are primarily metabolized by the liver [62].

- These drugs should be administered with extreme care to patients with age/gestational age under two months.
- Modifications of dosing should be based on response to treatment and on therapeutic drug monitoring.
- After six months of age, body surface area is a good basis for dosing, but dosing for drugs that are primarily metabolized by CYP2D6 and UDP should be based on weight.

In the future, it is possible that an individualized dose could be calculated by studying the activity and content of the phase I and phase II enzymes involved in the metabolism of the substance of interest.

The interindividual variability of pharmacokinetic data is high [6]. The variability is much greater in neonates and infants than in adults because all of the previously mentioned parameters influence each other and because processes change rapidly and individually.

References

1 Tayman C, Rayyan M, Allegaert K: Neonatal pharmacology: extensive interindividual variability despite limited size. J Pediatr Pharmacol Ther 2011;16: 170–184.

2 Hines RN: The ontogeny of drug metabolism enzymes and implications for adverse drug events. Pharmacol Ther 2008;118:250–267.

3 Anderson BJ, McKee AD, Holford NH: Size, myths and the clinical pharmacokinetics of analgesia in paediatric patients. Clin Pharmacokinet 1997;33: 313–327.

4 Hines RN, McCarver DG: The ontogeny of human drug-metabolizing enzymes: phase I oxidative enzymes. J Pharmacol Exp Ther 2002;300:355–360.

5 McCarver DG, Hines RN: The ontogeny of human drug-metabolizing enzymes: phase II conjugation enzymes and regulatory mechanisms. J Pharmacol Exp Ther 2002;300:361–366.

6 Alcorn J, McNamara PJ: Ontogeny of hepatic and renal systemic clearance pathways in infants: part I. Clin Pharmacokinet 2002;41:959–998.

7 de Wildt SN, Kearns GL, Leeder JS, van den Anker JN: Glucuronidation in humans. Pharmacogenetic and developmental aspects. Clin Pharmacokinet 1999;36:439–452.

8 Weiss CF, Glazko AJ, Weston JK: Chloramphenicol in the newborn infant. A physiologic explanation of its toxicity when given in excessive doses. N Engl J Med 1960;262:787–794.

9 Alam SN, Roberts RJ, Fischer LJ: Age-related differences in salicylamide and acetaminophen conjugation in man. J Pediatr 1977;90:130–135.

10 Kearns GL, Abdel-Rahman SM, Alander SW, Blowey DL, Leeder JS, Kauffman RE: Developmental pharmacology – drug disposition, action, and therapy in infants and children. N Engl J Med 2003;349: 1157–1167.

11 Nelson DR, Kamataki T, Waxman DJ, Guengerich FP, Estabrook RW, Feyereisen R, Gonzalez FJ, Coon MJ, Gunsalus IC, Gotoh O: The P450 superfamily: update on new sequences, gene mapping, accession numbers, early trivial names of enzymes, and nomenclature. DNA Cell Biol 1993;12:1–51.

12 Shimada T, Yamazaki H, Mimura M, Wakamiya N, Ueng YF, Guengerich FP, Inui Y: Characterization of microsomal cytochrome P450 enzymes involved in the oxidation of xenobiotic chemicals in human fetal liver and adult lungs. Drug Metab Dispos 1996;24: 515–522.

13 Cresteil T, Beaune P, Kremers P, Celier C, Guengerich FP, Leroux JP: Immunoquantification of epoxide hydrolase and cytochrome P-450 isozymes in fetal and adult human liver microsomes. Eur J Biochem 1985;151:345–350.

14 Allegaert K, Anderson BJ, Cossey V, Holford NH: Limited predictability of amikacin clearance in extreme premature neonates at birth. Br J Clin Pharmacol 2006;61:39–48.

15 Rane A: Phenotyping of drug metabolism in infants and children: potentials and problems. Pediatrics 1999;104:640–643.
16 de Wildt SN, Kearns GL, Leeder JS, van den Anker JN: Cytochrome P450 3A: ontogeny and drug disposition. Clin Pharmacokinet 1999;37:485–505.
17 Kivistö KT, Bookjans G, Fromm MF, Griese EU, Münzel P, Kroemer HK: Expression of CYP3A4, CYP3A5 and CYP3A7 in human duodenal tissue. Br J Clin Pharmacol 1996;42:387–389.
18 McKinnon RA, Burgess WM, Hall PM, Roberts-Thomson SJ, Gonzalez FJ, McManus ME: Characterisation of CYP3A gene subfamily expression in human gastrointestinal tissues. Gut 1995;36:259–267.
19 Watkins PB, Wrighton SA, Schuetz EG, Molowa DT, Guzelian PS: Identification of glucocorticoid-inducible cytochromes P-450 in the intestinal mucosa of rats and man. J Clin Invest 1987;80:1029–1036.
20 Nelson DR, Koymans L, Kamataki T, Stegeman JJ, Feyereisen R, Waxman DJ, Waterman MR, Gotoh O, Coon MJ, Estabrook RW, Gunsalus IC, Nebert DW: P450 superfamily: update on new sequences, gene mapping, accession numbers and nomenclature. Pharmacogenetics 1996;6:1–42.
21 Shimada T, Yamazaki H, Mimura M, Inui Y, Guengerich FP: Interindividual variations in human liver cytochrome P-450 enzymes involved in the oxidation of drugs, carcinogens and toxic chemicals: studies with liver microsomes of 30 Japanese and 30 Caucasians. J Pharmacol Exp Ther 1994;270:414–423.
22 Chiba M, Nshime JA, Lin JH: In vitro metabolism of indinavir in the human fetal liver microsomes. Drug Metab Dispos 1997;25:1219–1222.
23 Tateishi T, Nakura H, Asoh M, Watanabe M, Tanaka M, Kumai T, Takashima S, Imaoka S, Funae Y, Yabusaki Y, Kamataki T, Kobayashi S: A comparison of hepatic cytochrome P450 protein expression between infancy and postinfancy. Life Sci 1997;61:2567–2574.
24 Yang HY, Lee QP, Rettie AE, Juchau MR: Functional cytochrome P4503A isoforms in human embryonic tissues: expression during organogenesis. Mol Pharmacol 1994;46:922–928.
25 Inoue K, Inazawa J, Nakagawa H, Shimada T, Yamazaki H, Guengerich FP, Abe T: Assignment of the human cytochrome P-450 nifedipine oxidase gene (CYP3A4) to chromosome 7 at band q22.1 by fluorescence in situ hybridization. Jpn J Hum Genet 1992;37:133–138.
26 Komori M, Nishio K, Ohi H, Kitada M, Kamataki T: Molecular cloning and sequence analysis of cDNA containing the entire coding region for human fetal liver cytochrome P-450. J Biochem 1989;105:161–163.
27 Ohmori S, Nakasa H, Asanome K, Kurose Y, Ishii I, Hosokawa M, Kitada M: Differential catalytic properties in metabolism of endogenous and exogenous substrates among CYP3A enzymes expressed in COS-7 cells. Biochim Biophys Acta 1998;1380:297–304.
28 Kitada M, Kamataki T, Itahashi K, Rikihisa T, Kato R, Kanakubo Y: Purification and properties of cytochrome P-450 from homogenates of human fetal livers. Arch Biochem Biophys 1985;241:275–280.
29 Hines RN: Ontogeny of human hepatic cytochromes P450. J Biochem Mol Toxicol 2007;21:169–175.
30 Kolars JC, Lown KS, Schmiedlin-Ren P, Ghosh M, Fang C, Wrighton SA, Merion RM, Watkins PB: CYP3A gene expression in human gut epithelium. Pharmacogenetics 1994;4:247–259.
31 de Waziers I, Cugnenc PH, Yang CS, Leroux JP, Beaune PH: Cytochrome P 450 isoenzymes, epoxide hydrolase and glutathione transferases in rat and human hepatic and extrahepatic tissues. J Pharmacol Exp Ther 1990;253:387–394.
32 Hall SD, Thummel KE, Watkins PB, Lown KS, Benet LZ, Paine MF, Mayo RR, Turgeon DK, Bailey DG, Fontana RJ, Wrighton SA: Molecular and physical mechanisms of first-pass extraction. Drug Metab Dispos 1999;27:161–166.
33 Lang CC, Brown RM, Kinirons MT, Deathridge MA, Guengerich FP, Kelleher D, O'Briain DS, Ghishan FK, Wood AJ: Decreased intestinal CYP3A in celiac disease: reversal after successful gluten-free diet: a potential source of interindividual variability in first-pass drug metabolism. Clin Pharmacol Ther 1996; 59:41–46.
34 Schuetz JD, Beach DL, Guzelian PS: Selective expression of cytochrome P450 CYP3A mRNAs in embryonic and adult human liver. Pharmacogenetics 1994; 4:11–20.
35 Lacroix D, Sonnier M, Moncion A, Cheron G, Cresteil T: Expression of CYP3A in the human liver–evidence that the shift between CYP3A7 and CYP3A4 occurs immediately after birth. Eur J Biochem 1997; 247:625–634.
36 Greuet J, Pichard L, Bonfils C, Domergue J, Maurel PM: The fetal specific gene CYP3A7 is inducible by rifampicin in adult human hepatocytes in primary culture. Biochem Biophys Res Commun 1996;225: 689–694.
37 Hakkola J, Pasanen M, Purkunen R, Saarikoski S, Pelkonen O, Mäenpää J, Rane A, Raunio H: Expression of xenobiotic-metabolizing cytochrome P450 forms in human adult and fetal liver. Biochem Pharmacol 1994;48:59–64.
38 Lechevrel M, Casson AG, Wolf CR, Hardie LJ, Flinterman MB, Montesano R, Wild CP: Characterization of cytochrome P450 expression in human oesophageal mucosa. Carcinogenesis 1999;20:243–248.
39 Paine MF, Khalighi M, Fisher JM, Shen DD, Kunze KL, Marsh CL, Perkins JD, Thummel KE: Characterization of interintestinal and intraintestinal variations in human CYP3A-dependent metabolism. J Pharmacol Exp Ther 1997;283:552–562.

40 Wrighton SA, Stevens JC: The human hepatic cytochromes P450 involved in drug metabolism. Crit Rev Toxicol 1992;22:1–21.
41 Treluyer JM, Jacqz-Aigrain E, Alvarez F, Cresteil T: Expression of CYP2D6 in developing human liver. Eur J Biochem 1991;202:583–588.
42 Allegaert K, Anderson BJ, Verbesselt R, Debeer A, de Hoon J, Devlieger H, Van Den Anker JN, Tibboel D: Tramadol disposition in the very young: an attempt to assess in vivo cytochrome P-450 2D6 activity. Br J Anaesth 2005;95:231–239.
43 Allegaert K, Van den Anker JN, Debeer A, Cossey V, Verbesselt R, Tibboel D, Devlieger H, de Hoon J: Maturational changes in the in vivo activity of CYP3A4 in the first months of life. Int J Clin Pharmacol Ther 2006;44:303–308.
44 Allegaert K, Van den Anker JN, Verbesselt R, de Hoon J, Vanhole C, Tibboel D, Devlieger H: O-demethylation of tramadol in the first months of life. Eur J Clin Pharmacol 2005;61:837–842.
45 Wheeler CW, Wrighton SA, Guenthner TM: Detection of human lung cytochromes P450 that are immunochemically related to cytochrome P450IIE1 and cytochrome P450IIIA. Biochem Pharmacol 1992;44:183–187.
46 Hansson T, Tindberg N, Ingelman-Sundberg M, Köhler C: Regional distribution of ethanol-inducible cytochrome P450 IIE1 in the rat central nervous system. Neuroscience 1990;34:451–463.
47 Thummel KE, Kharasch ED, Podoll T, Kunze K: Human liver microsomal enflurane defluorination catalyzed by cytochrome P-450 2E1. Drug Metab Dispos 1993;21:350–357.
48 Raucy JL, Lasker JM, Lieber CS, Black M: Acetaminophen activation by human liver cytochromes P450IIE1 and P450IA2. Arch Biochem Biophys 1989;271:270–283.
49 Ekström G, von Bahr C, Ingelman-Sundberg M: Human liver microsomal cytochrome P-450IIE1. Immunological evaluation of its contribution to microsomal ethanol oxidation, carbon tetrachloride reduction and NADPH oxidase activity. Biochem Pharmacol 1989;38:689–693.
50 Vieira I, Sonnier M, Cresteil T: Developmental expression of CYP2E1 in the human liver. Hypermethylation control of gene expression during the neonatal period. Eur J Biochem 1996;238:476–483.
51 Smith M, Hopkinson DA, Harris H: Developmental changes and polymorphism in human alcohol dehydrogenase. Ann Hum Genet 1971;34:251–271.
52 Miyagi SJ, Collier AC: The development of UDP-glucuronosyltransferases 1A1 and 1A6 in the pediatric liver. Drug Metab Dispos 2011;39:912–919.
53 Bouwmeester NJ, Anderson BJ, Tibboel D, Holford NH: Developmental pharmacokinetics of morphine and its metabolites in neonates, infants and young children. Br J Anaesth 2004;92:208–217.
54 Kimland E, Nydert P, Odlind V, Bottiger Y, Lindemalm S: Paediatric drug use with focus on off-label prescriptions at Swedish hospitals – a nationwide study. Acta Paediatrica 2012;101:772–778.
55 Zuppa AF, Hammer GB, Barrett JS, Kenney BF, Kassir N, Mouksassi S, Royal MA: Safety and population pharmacokinetic analysis of intravenous acetaminophen in neonates, infants, children, and adolescents with pain or fever. J Pediatr Pharmacol Ther 2011;16: 246–261.
56 Palmer GM, Atkins M, Anderson BJ, Smith KR, Culnane TJ, McNally CM, Perkins EJ, Chalkiadis GA, Hunt RW: I.V. acetaminophen pharmacokinetics in neonates after multiple doses. Br J Anaesth 2008;101: 523–530.
57 van der Marel CD, Anderson BJ, van Lingen RA, Holford NH, Pluim MA, Jansman FG, van den Anker JN, Tibboel D: Paracetamol and metabolite pharmacokinetics in infants. Eur J Clin Pharmacol 2003; 59:243–251.
58 Ghanem CI, Ruiz ML, Villanueva SS, Luquita MG, Catania VA, Jones B, Bengochea LA, Vore M, Mottino AD: Shift from biliary to urinary elimination of acetaminophen-glucuronide in acetaminophen-pretreated rats. J Pharmacol Exp Ther 2005;315:987–995.
59 Allegaert K, de Hoon J, Verbesselt R, Vanhole C, Devlieger H, Tibboel D: Intra- and interindividual variability of glucuronidation of paracetamol during repeated administration of propacetamol in neonates. Acta Paediatr 2005;94:1273–1279.
60 Krumbiegel P, Domke S, Mörseburg B, Boehm G, Braun W: Maturation of hepatosomal mono-oxygenation and glucuronidation activities in pre- and full-term infants as studied using the [15N]methacetin urine test. Acta Paediatr 1997;86:1236–1240.
61 Kennedy M: Hormonal regulation of hepatic drug-metabolizing enzyme activity during adolescence. Clin Pharmacol Ther 2008;84:662–673.
62 Bartelink IH, Rademaker CM, Schobben AF, van den Anker JN: Guidelines on paediatric dosing on the basis of developmental physiology and pharmacokinetic considerations. Clin Pharmacokinet 2006;45: 1077–1097.

Synnöve Lindemalm
Astrid Lindgren Children's Hospital
Department for Quality and Safety
Karolinska University Hospital
SE–171 76 Stockholm (Sweden)
E-Mail synnove.lindemalm@karolinska.se

Mimouni FB, van den Anker JN (eds): Neonatal Pharmacology and Nutrition Update.
Pediatr Adolesc Med. Basel, Karger, 2015, vol 18, pp 13–27 (DOI: 10.1159/000364989)

How to Translate Pharmacokinetic Data into Dosing Recommendations

Elke H.J. Krekels[a, b] · Catherijne A.J. Knibbe[a, b] · Paula Pokorna[a, c] · Dick Tibboel[a]

[a]Intensive Care and Department of Pediatric Surgery, Erasmus MC – Sophia Children's Hospital, Rotterdam, The Netherlands; [b]Division of Pharmacology, Leiden Academic Center for Drug Research, Leiden University, Leiden, The Netherlands; [c]Intensive Care Department of Pediatrics, First Medical Faculty, Charles University, Prague, Czech Republic

Abstract

Pharmacotherapy in children is challenging due to limited knowledge of the influence of physiological changes on drug exposure and response. Differences in drug pharmacokinetics are often considered the main drivers of age-related differences in dose requirements in neonates and young infants. Pharmacokinetic parameters in these young children can be derived from a *'population analysis'* of drug concentration measurements in the blood at various time points after drug administration. A major advantage of performing a population analysis is that it allows investigations into between-subject variability. Patient characteristics that can describe patterns in the variability of pharmacokinetic parameters can be used to predict these pharmacokinetic parameters in other patients within the same population. The distribution volume of a drug is the main driver of peak concentrations, whereas drug clearance is the driver of steady state concentrations. Information on how these parameters differ between individuals within a given population therefore allows clinicians to determine drug doses that correct for these differences, leading to the same exposure for each patient. The patient characteristics that predict the variability in pharmacokinetic parameters are called covariates, and the mathematical equations describing their relationship with the pharmacokinetic parameters can be used as the basis for evidence-based pediatric dosing recommendations.

In the pediatric population, which ranges from newborn infants with extreme low birth weight up to adolescents, many ontogenetic changes result in increased variability in drug effects compared to the effects in adults [1, 2]. In addition to marked increases in body size, there are significant changes in the expression and function of drug-metabolizing enzymes and transporters. In addition, differences in cardiac output and blood flow influence the perfusion of drug-clearing organs, and differences in the acid-base balance and the concentration and composition of drug-binding plasma proteins and other blood components may influence concentrations of unbound drug in the blood. Furthermore, as the amounts of total body water and extracellular water decrease with age, the relative size of the organs changes, as does the body composition. Moreover, the pH in various parts of the gastro-intestinal-tract in the pediatric population is different from that in adults, as are gastric emptying time and intestinal motility. All of these factors may alter drug exposure in pediatric patients. Likewise, developmental changes may influence pharmacodynamics and affect the variability of the pediatric drug response. For example, changes in the function and relative number of receptors and target proteins can alter a patient's sensitivity to a drug, while for drugs with targets outside the circulatory system, the time-course of the drug's effects can be altered due to changes in the distribution of the drug from the blood to the site of action. In addition to these issues, disease status may affect the physiological system and the physiological feedback mechanisms, thus making diseases that are unique to the pediatric population or diseases that progress differently in children and adults unique contributors to the variability of pediatric drug response. Particularly in neonates, numerous and profound physiological changes occur in quick succession and within a short period of time. Pharmacotherapy for these youngest patients is therefore accompanied by major challenges, and increased knowledge about the influence of these physiological changes on pharmacology is therefore particularly relevant. Unfortunately, systematic approaches to improve this situation are scarce in the literature.

With the current lack of evidence-based dosing recommendations, empiric drug dosing in children is very common. The number of pediatric patients receiving at least one off-label or unlicensed drug was reported to range between 80 and 93% in neonatal intensive care units, between 36 and 100% in general pediatric wards, and between 3.3 and 56% in the ambulatory setting [3]. When evidence-based dosing recommendations are lacking, pediatric drug doses are often empirically derived from adult doses using linear extrapolation based on body weight, meaning that a child with half the body weight of an adult receives half the adult drug dose. Because this practice is known to fail to provide suitable drug doses over the entire pediatric age range, the amount that is prescribed per kilogram of body weight is often adjusted for different age groups, especially for the youngest patients. For example, consider vancomycin: for children between 1 and 18 months of age, 40 mg/kg/day divided into three doses is recommended, whereas for neonates between 1 and 4 weeks of age, 30 mg/kg/day is divided into three doses, and in neonates younger than 1 week of age, the recommended dose is further reduced to 20 mg/kg/day divided into 2 doses [4]. Dosing recommendations such as these often evolve over years of clinical experience and are sometimes formalized in (national) pediatric formularies [4, 5]. While these consensus-based dosing recommendations may reduce the risk of under- or overdosing patients, they still do not provide the level of scientific evidence that is obligatory for drug labeling in adults. This situation is highly undesirable, as suboptimal drug dosing may lead to unnecessary therapy failure or to overdosing, which may cause serious side effects and even fatalities.

Instead of empiric body weight-based dose adjustments, pediatric drug dosing recommendations should be based on a thorough understanding of the pharmacokinetics and pharmacodynamics of a drug in children. This understanding will allow optimization of the risk/benefit ratio by creating a balance between minimal drug exposure and maximum efficacy and safety. To improve pediatric drug dosing, it is therefore essential to study the influence of developmental changes in children on drug pharmacokinetics, including absorption, distribution, metabolism and elimination, as well as the influence of developmental changes on drug pharmacodynamics, including effect site distribution, target activation, and signal transduction. Additionally, it is important that developmental changes in pharmacokinetics are considered in the context of all other sources of variability in drug pharmacokinetics, such as demographic, genetic, environmental, and disease-related factors.

Despite the fact that a combination of pharmacokinetic and pharmacodynamic processes is responsible for drug effects, most studies in pediatric clinical pharmacology have hitherto focused on the developmental changes in drug pharmacokinetics, which will also be the focus of this chapter. Indeed, for many drugs, the developmental differences in drug clearance (the pharmacokinetic parameter that is the main driver of drug exposure) are thought to be the major causes of age-dependent differences in dose requirements [6]. The implicit assumption in these cases is that the pharmacodynamics of those drugs remains constant within the pediatric population. This assumption is acceptable when (1) the underlying pathophysiological processes are similar throughout the population; (2) based on the mechanism of action, the exposure-effect relationship can be assumed independent of age; and (3) the same clinical endpoints for treatment are used throughout the population.

This does not imply that conducting studies of pediatric pharmacokinetics is not important for drugs that do not meet these three criteria. The influence of developmental changes on the pharmacokinetics of these drugs may still be large, particularly in very young individuals. In these cases, drug treatment can already be improved by accounting for the differences in pharmacokinetics. Subsequent research on the pharmacodynamics of these drugs may further improve the dosing recommendation by revealing age-appropriate target concentrations in blood. In these investigations, knowledge of drug pharmacokinetics is also important because this knowledge will be the basis for pharmacodynamic studies.

Pharmacokinetic Studies in Neonates

Pharmacokinetic studies require drug concentrations to be measured in a biological tissue (usually blood or serum) at different time points after drug dosing. In neonates, this testing provides a unique set of challenges regarding ethical, legal, and practical constraints.

Because neonates cannot consent to participate in clinical studies, it is unethical (and in most countries illegal) to perform studies in healthy neonates. This restricts the potential study population to individuals requiring medical treatment. Moreover, these infants can only be included in a study after written informed consent is obtained from both parents and/or legal guardians. Compared to the adult population, the number of neonates is relatively small, while the heterogeneity in this population is large. Body weight alone may, for example, differ by up to a factor of ten between a 500-g premature neonate and a 5-kg term newborn at day 30 of life. By restricting pharmacokinetic studies to patients, the number of potential study subjects is further limited, while the heterogeneity of the population is further increased because of differences in the nature and the severity of the illness. In addition, multiple drug use (polypharmacy) in most of these patients may introduce drug-drug interactions in pharmacokinetic and pharmacodynamics processes. Finally, as most studies need to be performed within the routine medical care of these patients, drug dosing cannot always adhere to a stringent study design because most drugs need to be clinically titrated to individual medical needs, a process that is guided by both the efficacy and potential side effects of the drug.

Practical constraints for pharmacokinetic studies in neonates lie in the small blood volume of these patients, which limits the volume and number of blood samples that can be obtained from a single patient. In most countries, the total amount of blood that is allowed to be taken from neonates for research purposes is less than 3% of the circulating volume. Additionally, without an indwelling arterial line, arterial blood sampling for the sole purpose of pharmacokinetic studies is often not allowed. In these cases, blood sample collection cannot adhere to a strict predetermined schedule and must coincide with clinical care procedures that require arterial blood sampling. Before this so-called opportunistic sampling can be introduced as an alternative method of harvesting blood for pharmacokinetic studies, the presence of a well-defined infrastructure that allows for this type of sample processing is important. Modern technologies for pharmacokinetic sampling (e.g., dried blood spots, saliva) and sensitive sample analysis (e.g., LC-MS or electrophoresis) may further facilitate pharmacokinetic studies in neonates by overcoming some of the practical limitations.

Pharmacokinetic Data Analysis

In a pharmacokinetic data analysis, the drug concentrations measured in blood or serum at various time intervals after dosing are used to determine the values of parameters such as clearance, distribution volume, and absorption rate. This is performed by searching for a set of parameter values that result in a concentration-time profile that describes the observed concentrations well.

The standard two-stage approach to determining pharmacokinetic drug parameters in a population relies first on determining the values of the individual parameters. This is performed by obtaining a large amount of concentration-time information from each patient followed by determining the mean and standard deviation of each parameter. This approach is difficult with neonates, not only because a relatively large number of samples is required from each patient but also because the samples need to be obtained according to a stringent study design to ensure similar drug dosing and blood sampling in each individual. Additionally, this approach yields only one single point estimate (mean value) for each pharmacokinetic parameter for the overall study population and a single measure of variability (standard deviation) within this population. Using this approach, different sources of variability, such as between-subject variability and measurement error, cannot be identified. Moreover, because only one parameter value is obtained for the overall population, developmental patterns in the pediatric population can only be investigated by stratifying patients into age groups, quantifying pharmacokinetic parameters within each age group per kilogram body weight (e.g., ml/min/kg for clearance), and then describing the trends in the mean parameter values for each group. This process makes any findings on maturation patterns dependent on how the patients were stratified into age groups.

In the past few decades, more advanced, computer-intensive approaches have become available for the analysis of neonatal pharmacokinetic data. *'Population modeling'*, also known as *'non-linear mixed effect modeling'*, is now the preferred tool for the analysis of pharmacokinetic data in neonates. In population modeling, each individual is regarded a constituent of the overall population, while still taking into account that different data originate from different patients. By analyzing the population as a whole, fewer blood samples are required per individual, limiting the burden on individual patients. Additionally, the population modeling approach supports the simultaneous analysis of dense data (many observations per patient), sparse data (few observations per patient), and/or unbalanced data (many observations for some patients and few for others, or observations at different time points for each individual). This approach allows the analysis of data obtained during routine clinical practice with high variability in drug dosing and blood sampling; it also allows the pooling of (historic) data from studies with different designs.

The major advantage of the population-based approach in deriving dosing recommendations is that between-subject variability can be distinguished from other sources of variability, such as measurement error. Population models therefore yield not only one parameter value for the overall population but also a value (i.e., a posthoc parameter) for each individual within the population, even when a certain parameter value cannot be derived from the data obtained from an individual patient. This is relevant because it allows for investigations into the patterns of between-subject variability, as some patient characteristics may explain at least part of the variability between subjects. If, for example, the distribution volume of a drug is known to increase in patients with higher body weight, then knowing the body weight of a patient allows the clinician to make a better, more-informed prediction of that patient's distribution volume for that drug. Patient characteristics that can be used to describe and thereby predict individual differences in pharmacokinetic parameter values are called covariates. Covariates may have many different origins, such as demographic factors (e.g., age, gender, race), (patho)physiological factors (e.g., organ function, hemodynamics, disease status), genetics (e.g., rapid or slow metabolizer phenotype), or environmental factors (e.g., concomitant therapy). The covariates in the pharmacokinetic model of a drug can serve as the basis for evidence-based, individualized drug dosing recommendations.

Population Pharmacokinetic Model Development

The word 'mixed' in 'non-linear mixed effects modeling' (another name for population modeling), refers to the modeling of a mixture of so-called 'fixed effects' and 'random effects'. Fixed effects are described in a structural model (e.g., a one- or two-compartment model to describe a mono- or bi-exponential decline in drug concentration over time). The random effects quantify the variability that is not explained by the fixed effects and may include both between-subject variability and measurement error.

The development of a population pharmacokinetic model or a non-linear mixed effects model is performed in three steps: (1) development of a structural model that describes the time-course of drug concentrations as a fixed effect; (2) development of a stochastic model that describes and quantifies the various sources of variability as random effects; (3) development of a covariate model that describes the relationship between patient characteristics and a given structural model parameter.

As these three models are interrelated, the choice of the structural and stochastic models may affect the choice of the covariate model and *vice versa*. The process of finding a model that adequately describes the data is thus an elaborate task in which model building, checking, and refining are performed in several steps.

In addition to identifying patient characteristics (covariates) that describe and thereby predict between-subject variability in specific pharmacokinetic parameters, a covariate analysis also aims to define the mathematical equations that best describe this relationship. For example, when the distribution volume of a drug in one patient with twice the body weight of a second patient is double the distribution volume of the second patient, the relationship between body weight and distribution volume is said to be linear and is described by a linear equation:

$$V_i = V_p * BW_i. \qquad (1)$$

Equation 1 states that the distribution volume of a specific individual (V_i) is equal to a certain constant (which is often referred to as the population value for that parameter (V_p), the value of which does not change within a population) multiplied by the body weight of the individual (BW_i).

More complex equations are needed to describe more complex relationships. For example, when doubling the patient body weight yields an increase in clearance that is either more than twice as high or less than twice as high, an exponential equation may be used:

$$CL_i = CL_p * BW_i^{\,a} \tag{2}$$

Equation 2 states that the clearance for a specific individual (CL_i) depends on a certain population constant for that parameter (CL_p) multiplied by the individual's body weight (BW_i) raised to the power of 'a'. The value of 'a' in equation 2 describes the shape of the relationship. A value of 'a' that is greater than 1 describes a situation in which doubling the body weight yields more than double the individual clearance, whereas a value of 'a' that is less than 1 describes a situation in which doubling the body weight yields less than twice the individual clearance.

The influence of developmental changes in childhood on drug pharmacokinetic parameters is usually explored using body size and/or age as covariates. However, one must be careful when using 2 variables that are strongly correlated with each other (such as weight and age) as covariates because this may introduce a problem of collinearity, thereby making the prediction equation unstable. Size is often parameterized using body weight, although measures such as fat free mass or body surface area have also been used. In neonates and young children, age may be parameterized using, for example, postmenstrual age, gestational age or postnatal age. Covariate model building in neonates and children can be performed using one of two approaches.

The first approach is based on 'allometric scaling' [7]. In this approach, body weight (or another measure reflecting body size) is included in the covariate model in two different equations. Without confirming that these equations actually describe the individual parameter values well, body weight is included as a covariate in a linear relationship for distribution volume (equation 1) and in an exponential relationship with an exponent of 0.75 for clearance (equation 2, with the value of 'a' being set as 0.75). If these functions do not describe individual distribution volumes and clearances well, additional age-based functions of various forms are included in the model to improve the description. After body weight and age are included in the covariate model, the influence of other possible covariates (e.g., organ function) may be investigated. The application of allometric scaling in pediatric pharmacokinetics is controversial, as the theoretical basis and experimental evidence supporting this approach are weak [8, 9].

The second approach, known as 'systematic covariate analysis', investigates the influence of body weight and age in the same way as any other available covariate. Each potentially relevant covariate (e.g., body weight and age as well as demographic, genetic, and disease-related factors) is evaluated in a systematic manner, and covariates are only included in the covariate model when the resulting model significantly improves the description of the concentration-time data by improving the description of the individual parameter estimates [10]. Using a covariate model developed with this approach ensures that the model is always supported by the experimental data. By not placing preconceptions regarding the influence of body weight and age on pediatric pharmacokinetics into the covariate model, this approach may lead to unexpected results.

For example, it was found that in children between the age of one month and 17 years, the influence of disease state on midazolam clearance was greater than the influence of developmental changes. In the first month of life, the influence of developmental changes on midazolam clearance was more pronounced; nevertheless, the significant influence of disease state persisted. Not taking into account the disease state for critically ill neonates on midazolam treatment may therefore result in serious overdosing of these patients [11]. The impact of disease state or treatment modality on the pharmacokinetics of drugs has received little attention. However, there are additional factors that are known to influence drug pharmacokinetics in neonates and young children that should be taken into account together with developmental changes when determining drug doses for these patients. Examples in the literature include therapeutic hypothermia [12], ECMO treatment [13] and different types of cardiac surgery [14].

How are Pharmacokinetic Parameters Used for Dosing Recommendations?

A drug's concentration at the site of action is the main determinant of drug effect. For drugs whose site of action (e.g., receptor or target protein) is in the blood circulation or in fast-equilibrating tissue (e.g., tissues in which the drug concentrations closely follow the changes in drug concentration in blood), the concentration-time profile of that drug in the blood can be considered to be driving the drug effects. For systemically administered drugs whose site of action is in a tissue that equilibrates slowly with blood (e.g., due to poor perfusion) or in tissue that is protected by a barrier that slows down the equilibration between the drug concentration in the blood and in the tissue (e.g., the brain), the situation is more complex. However, the concentrations of these drugs in the bloodstream are not completely uninformative because after accounting for the delay in equilibration, the blood concentrations may still be predictive of the drug effect. In pharmacokinetic models, the concentration-time profile of a drug in blood that results from the absorption, distribution, metabolism and elimination processes is mathematically described using parameters such as *clearance, distribution volume* and *absorption rate constant.*

It can generally be said that with intravenous drug administration, the distribution volume of a drug mainly determines the peak concentration. Therefore, knowledge of how the distribution volume of a drug differs between patients is important for deriving recommendations for loading doses of this drug (e.g., induction of anesthesia with propofol), or for deriving recommendations for drugs with a mechanism of action that mainly relies on peak concentrations (e.g., the systemic treatment of bacterial infections with gentamicin or with other aminoglycosides). As such, if the variability in distribution volume between individuals for a given drug is best described by a linear body weight-based equation (equation 1), the loading doses for this drug should be calculated per kilogram of body weight (e.g., in mg/kg).

Steady state drug concentrations, by contrast, are solely determined by drug clearance. Therefore, knowing how clearance of a drug differs between patients is of importance for determining recommendations for repeated doses or continuous infusions. Thus, continuous infusions of a drug whose clearance increases exponentially with body weight to the power of 0.8 (equation 2 with the value of 'a' = 0.8) should be dosed in mg/kg$^{0.8}$/h.

Because a population analysis does not require stratification of patients by age groups to describe the influence of developmental changes on pharmacokinetic parameters, covariate relationships can often be defined with a continuous equation. This implies that one equation may describe or predict drug clearance for the entire study population. The dosing recommendation derived from this equation can therefore also be expressed as a single algorithm; this avoids dosing issues that may occur in patients at the extremes of intervals to which current dosing recommendations are often applied. In the example of vancomycin, for example, it may be difficult for a physician to decide whether to give a dose of 30 mg/kg/day (recommended for patients between 1 and 4 weeks) or a dose of 40 mg/kg/day (recommended for patients between 1 and 18 months) to a patient who is 29 days old. Furthermore, if a dose of 30 mg/kg/day is selected, at what day should the dose be increased to 40 mg/kg/day? On the other hand, a disadvantage of some of the continuous covariate relationships obtained from population models is that these models may yield complex dosing algorithms, such as dosing in mg/kg$^{0.8}$/h. Such dosing recommendations may be difficult to implement in clinical practice. However, it is important to note that dosing recommendations should be as simple as possible, not simpler. To avoid miscalculation of a drug dose for a specific patient at the bedside, close involvement of the hospital pharmacist may be required for patient care in addition to the use of dosing tables or electronic prescription systems [15].

Finally, it must be emphasized that the findings obtained from pediatric pharmacokinetic population models and the dosing recommendations derived therefore cannot be used for extrapolation outside the studied population. This is because, particularly in the very young, many changes occur in a short time frame, and the net influence of these numerous changes on the pharmacokinetics of drugs in unstudied patients cannot be predicted with any certainty. It has, for example, been reported that the influence of developmental changes on the clearance of propofol can be described throughout the pediatric age range by a body weight-based exponential equation with an exponent that depends on body weight (equation 2, with the value of 'a' changing with body weight). The change in the value of the exponent, and thus the change in the maturation profile of clearance, are highly non-linear and is most pronounced in early childhood [16].

How to Develop Evidence-Based Dosing Recommendations: from Start to Finish

When developing evidence-based dosing recommendations that correct for differences in the pharmacokinetics of drugs, four important steps can be identified:

(1) Optimal Trial Design

The outcome of every study depends on a good design. The development of population pharmacokinetic studies is based on concentration-time data. As mentioned above, in neonates, it is not always possible to dose drugs or to sample blood according to a stringent protocol, although some flexibility is often possible within the normal care of these patients. A good study, therefore, starts with simulating the outcome of the designed study using a population model. Such simulations require information about the drug's pharmacokinetics as input, which is generally not available to studies for which obtaining this information is the objective. However, in many cases, there may already be some information available in the literature that permits educated guesses about the pharmacokinetics of a specific drug in neonates. Recent advances in '*physiologically based pharmacokinetic modeling*' have proven to be very useful in obtaining estimates for pharmacokinetic parameter values for this purpose [17].

It should be noted that the quality of a simulation depends on the quality of the assumptions that are put into it. In situations where the uncertainty of the assumptions is very high, the influence of the assumptions on the study outcome may be tested in a sensitivity analysis in which multiple scenarios are simulated (e.g., scenarios with different drug clearance values for neonates) to evaluate how each scenario would affect the study outcome. In the end, these simulations do not provide exact information, but they do provide guidance with regards to time frames. Generally, blood samples obtained around the peak of a concentration-time curve contain information that is highly useful for determining pharmacokinetic parameters involved in absorption processes and drug distribution, whereas blood samples taken at the tail of the profile contain more information about drug clearance. Knowing the approximate shape of the concentration-time curve will provide some information about the best times to obtain blood samples that will yield the most information with the least amount of sampling; it may also prevent unnecessary costs to and burdens on patients by avoiding blood sampling at time points when concentrations are too low to be detected.

(2) Development of the Population Pharmacokinetic Population Model

Based on the data obtained from a pharmacokinetic study, a pharmacokinetic population model, including a covariate model, can be developed as described in the section on pharmacokinetic data analysis. When the number of patients and samples in a study are limited, these data may be combined with data from other available sources. In some cases, it has even been possible to develop a population pharmacokinetic model solely on the basis of information obtained during routine clinical practice, for example, for therapeutic drug monitoring. It is important to note, however, that not all data can be pooled for a population pharmacokinetic analysis. These analyses require detailed records of the actual amount and time of each drug dose and the actual time of blood sampling; protocol times alone do not suffice for this purpose. In addition, accurate information about potentially important covariates is necessary. To this end, the execution of pharmacokinetic studies in neonates warrants a well-organized and solid infrastructure.

It should also be emphasized that there is an increased risk of drawing the wrong conclusions in an analysis, particularly when models are based on sparse data (i.e., a limited amount of information per patient), which is often the case with studies of neonates and young infants. This could have far-reaching consequences when clinical decisions or dosing recommendations are based on parameter values and covariate relationships obtained in such an analysis. Proper evaluation of the descriptive and predictive properties of the model is therefore essential. Evaluation of population models using the data that were used to develop the model is called internal validation. Various tools for the validation of population models are available, although many of them require special attention when applied to models for the pediatric population [18].

(3) External Validation of the Population Pharmacokinetic Population Model

A famous quote by George E.P. Box states that *'all models are wrong, but some are useful'*. When using a pharmacokinetic population model to derive dosing recommendations, it should be confirmed that the model is *'useful'* for this purpose. The best way to determine the usefulness of a population pharmacokinetic model for deriving dosing recommendations is to perform a so-called external validation. The results of the external validation should show whether a model can accurately predict pharmacokinetic parameters and/or drug concentrations using independent data (i.e., data that were not used to develop the model) obtained in the same population. Because external data for neonates may be scarce, another option that can be applied with datasets that are sufficiently large is the use of subsets of the dataset. In this approach, a portion of the data is used for model development (usually approximately 2/3 of the data), and the remaining data are used for external validation. In either case, it is important to ascertain that the patients in the external dataset provide a good representation of the patients in the original internal dataset. This can be performed by ensuring that the range of covariates in the external dataset sufficiently covers the range of covariates in the internal dataset. Without proper internal and external validation, a model cannot be regarded as a safe and reliable source for clinical decision making or for deriving dosing recommendations.

(4) Prospective Clinical Trial

Before the dosing recommendations that correct for differences in pharmacokinetics can be used in clinical practice, they should be prospectively evaluated in a clinical trial to ascertain that the model-derived dosing recommendation achieves the desired pharmacological effect. Blood concentrations can be expected to differ from the known (study) situation, particularly when a new dosing recommendation deviates from the dosing scheme used in a clinical study or from commonly used consensus-based recommendations. This may cause unexpected drug exposure, particularly in a situation with non-linear kinetics (e.g., saturation of elimination pathways), thereby causing unexpected responses or drug-related side effects. Moreover, when new dosing recommendations are based on a pharmacokinetic analysis and without considering the pharmacodynamics or the drug safety, differences in drug exposure resulting from the new dosing recommendation may also lead to unexpected responses. However, when a prospective study confirms that a model-derived recommendation yields the expected exposure without negatively affecting drug response or safety, it can be published as an evidence-based pediatric dosing recommendation.

The approach described above has been illustrated using morphine. A pharmacokinetic population model was developed based on morphine and metabolite concentration data in preterm and term neonates up to children of three years of age. According to this model, the changes in morphine glucuronidation clearance in this population are best described using a body weight-based exponential equation with an exponent of approximately 1.5 (equation 2 with the value of '*a*' = 1.44). In addition, glucuronidation was found to be reduced by 50% in neonates younger than ten days, irrespective of the gestational age. This reduction was expressed by a value of CL_p (equation 2) for young neonates that was approximately half the value of that for older children [19]. Based on these results, a clinical trial was conducted in which neonates younger than ten days received continuous morphine infusions for postoperative analgesia at an initial rate of 2.5 $\mu g/kg^{1.5}/h$, while older children up to the age of one year received 5 $\mu g/kg^{1.5}/h$. Compared to the traditional morphine infusion rate of 10 μg/kg/h, this meant a dose reduction of up to 75% for very young and lightweight neonates and a dose increase of up to 150% for the older patients. In this study, an age-appropriate protocol was used to adjust morphine consumption to individual patients' needs. From the actual morphine consumption, it could be concluded that the reduced morphine dose in the very young yielded sufficient analgesia, whereas a substantial need for rescue medication remained in the older patients [20]. Because the dosing algorithm used in this study corrects for differences in pharmacokinetics between the younger and older patients, the difference in the need for rescue mediation is most likely the result of differences in the pharmacodynamics of morphine in these groups. Determining age-appropriate target concentrations for morphine and its metabolites in the bloodstream and adjusting the dose such that these target concentrations are obtained may therefore further improve morphine dosing in this young population. However, adjusting morphine doses for differences in pharmacokinetics already showed an ability to reduce overdosing in the very young while simultaneously reducing the risk of exposure to ineffective doses in older patients.

Future Perspectives

It would require a tremendous amount of resources to develop and thoroughly validate pediatric pharmacokinetic and/or pharmacodynamic population models for each individual drug in neonates and children in the systematic manner described above. Hence, novel approaches are currently being investigated to limit the amount of resources required and to expedite the development of population pharmacokinetic models for the pediatric population.

A promising approach is based on the hypothesis that pediatric covariate relationships for drug elimination describe *system-specific* properties rather than *drug-specific* properties and can therefore be directly extrapolated from one drug to another drug that shares a common elimination pathway. In other words, it can be expected that the influence of changes in liver size, liver blood flow, and the expression and function of specific metabolic enzymes in neonates is the same for two different drugs that are metabolized by the same hepatic isoenzyme. In that case, it should be possible to use the same covariate relationship for clearance for both drugs, which in turn would lead to the same dosing algorithm (e.g., $mg/kg^{0.8}/h$) for both drugs. The absolute rate of clearance is a drug-specific property influenced by, among other properties, the affinity of the drug for a particular enzyme; therefore, the absolute dose may differ (e.g., 15 $mg/kg^{0.8}/h$ for a drug with lower affinity and 25 $mg/kg^{0.8}/h$ for a drug with higher affinity). However, determining absolute clearance in a population requires fewer data and fewer resources and can be performed faster than determining the full covariate relationship of the influence of developmental changes on drug clearance. This approach, which can be considered a combination of population pharmacokinetic modeling and physiologically based pharmacokinetic modeling, might therefore considerably expedite the development of evidence-based pediatric dosing recommendations.

The above hypothesis is supported by findings for the glucuronidation of UGT2B7 substrates [21] and for the renal clearance of aminoglycosides [22]. However, the broader applicability to situations with different rate-limiting steps in clearance mechanisms and drug clearance through multiple routes, as well as the applicability to other pharmacokinetic processes such as absorption, requires further investigation. Because misspecification of covariate relationships in this approach may be perpetuated to other drugs, the proper validation of the pediatric population models and the covariate relationships in these models becomes even more important. On the other hand, with this methodology, the development and validation of pediatric covariate models for specific pharmacokinetics processes does not have to be based on data only for the same drugs; it may also be based on data for different drugs that share the same elimination pathway. The ability to use more data may improve the precision of pediatric covariate models while simultaneously reducing the information required to evaluate drugs that have not been studied in children but are eliminated through a pathway that has already been studied in this population. Therefore, the development of more general '*systems models*' that contain pediatric covariate relationships that describe and predict the influence of developmental changes on drug clearance through a specific elimination pathway may provide a future basis for evidence-based dosing guidelines for existing and new drugs in neonates.

References

1 Kearns GL, Abdel-Rahman SM, Alander SW, Blowey DL, Leeder JS, Kauffman RE: Developmental pharmacology – drug disposition, action, and therapy in infants and children. N Engl J Med 2003;349:1157–1167.

2 Stephenson T: How children's responses to drugs differ from adults. Br J Clin Pharmacol 2005;59:670–673.

3 Cuzzolin L, Atzei A, Fanos V: Off-label and unlicensed prescribing for newborns and children in different settings: a review of the literature and a consideration about drug safety. Expert Opin Drug Saf 2006;5:703–718.

4 www.kinderformularium.nl.

5 www.bnf.org.

6 Alcorn J, McNamara PJ: Ontogeny of hepatic and renal systemic clearance pathways in infants: part I. Clin Pharmacokinet 2002;41:959–998.

7 Anderson BJ, Allegaert K, Holford NH: Population clinical pharmacology of children: modelling covariate effects. Eur J Pediatr 2006;165:819–829.

8 Agutter PS, Tuszynski JA: Analytic theories of allometric scaling. J Exp Biol 2011;214:1055–1062.

9 Mahmood I: Application of fixed exponent 0.75 to the prediction of human drug clearance: an inaccurate and misleading concept. Drug Metabol Drug Interact 2009;24:57–81.

10 De Cock RF, Piana C, Krekels EH, Danhof M, Allegaert K, Knibbe CA: The role of population PKPD modelling in paediatric clinical research. Eur J Clin Pharmacol 2011;67:5–16.

11 Ince I, de Wildt SN, Wang C, Peeters MY, Burggraaf J, Jacqz-Aigrain E, van den Anker JN, Tibboel D, Danhof M, Knibbe CA: A novel maturation function for clearance of the cytochrome P450 3A substrate midazolam from preterm neonates to adults. Clin Pharmacokinet 2013;52:555–565.

12 Zanelli S, Buck M, Fairchild K: Physiologic and pharmacologic considerations for hypothermia therapy in neonates. J Perinatol 2011;31:377–386.

13 Wildschut ED, Ahsman MJ, Houmes RJ, Pokorna P, de Wildt SN, Mathot RA, Tibboel D: Pharmacotherapy in neonatal and pediatric extracorporeal membrane oxygenation (ECMO). Curr Drug Metab 2012;13:767–777.

14 Dagan O, Klein J, Bohn D, Barker G, Koren G: Morphine pharmacokinetics in children following cardiac surgery: effects of disease and inotropic support. J Cardiothorac Vasc Anesth 1993;7:396–398.

15 Knibbe CA, Danhof M: Individualized dosing regimens in children based on population PKPD modelling: are we ready for it? Int J Pharm 2011;415:9–14.

16 Wang C, Peeters MY, Allegaert K, Blussé van Oud-Alblas HJ, Krekels EH, Tibboel D, Danhof M, Knibbe CA: A bodyweight-dependent allometric exponent for scaling clearance across the human life-span. Pharm Res 2012;29:1570–1581.

17 Johnson TN, Rostami-Hodjegan A, Tucker GT: Prediction of the clearance of eleven drugs and associated variability in neonates, infants and children. Clin Pharmacokinet 2006;45:931–956.

18 Krekels EH, van Hasselt JG, Tibboel D, Danhof M, Knibbe CA: Systematic evaluation of the descriptive and predictive performance of paediatric morphine population models. Pharm Res 2011;28:797–811.

19 Knibbe CA, Krekels EH, van den Anker JN, DeJongh J, Santen GW, van Dijk M, Simons SH, van Lingen RA, Jacqz-Aigrain EM, Danhof M, Tibboel D: Morphine glucuronidation in preterm neonates, infants and children younger than 3 years. Clin Pharmacokinet 2009;48:371–385.

20 Krekels EHJ, Tibboel D, De Wildt SN, Ceelie I, Dahan A, van Dijk M, Danhof M, Knibbe CAJ: Evidence-based morphine dosing for postoperative neonates and infants. Clin Pharmacokinet 2014;53: 553–563.

21 Krekels EHJ, Neely M, Panoilia E, Tibboel D, Capparelli E, Danhof M, Mirochnick M, Knibbe CAJ: From pediatric covariate model to semiphysiological function for maturation: part I–extrapolation of a covariate model from morphine to zidovudine. CPT Pharmacometrics Syst Pharmacol 2012;1:e9.

22 De Cock RFW, Allegaert K, Sherwin CMT, Nielsen EL, de Hoog M, van den Anker JN, Danhof M, Knibbe CAJ: A neonatal amikacin covariate model can be used to predict ontogeny of other drugs eliminated through glomerular filtration in neonates. Pharm Res 2014;31:754–767.

Dick Tibboel, MD, PhD
Intensive Care and Department of Pediatric Surgery
Erasmus MC-Sophia Childrens Hospital
Wytemaweg 80
NL–3015 CN Rotterdam (The Netherlands)
E-Mail d.tibboel@erasmusmc.nl

Mimouni FB, van den Anker JN (eds): Neonatal Pharmacology and Nutrition Update.
Pediatr Adolesc Med. Basel, Karger, 2015, vol 18, pp 28–40 (DOI: 10.1159/000364991)

Pharmacovigilance in Neonatal Intensive Care

Mark A. Turner • Helen Hill

Department of Women's and Children's Health, Institute of Translational Medicine, University of Liverpool, Liverpool, UK

Abstract

It is essential to balance the benefits and risks of the use of medicines in critically ill newborn infants with the primary goal not to harm (primum non nocere). To prevent drug-related harm it is important to avoid both medical errors that arise when medicines are not used as intended and adverse drug reactions (ADRs) that arise when medicines are used as intended. This chapter focuses on neonatal pharmacovigilance as an essential part of neonatal clinical care and provides several clear guidelines to prevent or minimize ADRs. Two main steps are proposed: 1) minimizing risk by following good prescribing practice and 2) when a concern or suspicion has been raised, taking a systematic approach. Both steps are systematically discussed and divided in many smaller steps for a logical approach. Furthermore, specific attention is given to specific features of pharmacovigilance in the neonatal intensive care unit (NICU) and during clinical trials. In the NICU settings the major difficulty in distinguishing between observed harms arising from the medical treatment or from underlying medical conditions is illustrated whereas for the clinical trials settings the differences in pharmacovigilance during early phase drug studies versus studies with well-known medicines is clarified. At the end the potential risks of excipients as culprits of ADRs are discussed.

Introduction

Medicines can cause harm as well as do good. It is essential to balance the harms and benefits of medicines. Given the large numbers of medicines to which sick babies are exposed, pharmacovigilance is at the heart of practice and research in neonatal units. According to the WHO, 'Pharmacovigilance is defined as the science and activities relating to the detection, assessment, understanding and prevention of adverse effects or any other drug-related problem' [1].

Several activities are involved in this definition. Many of these activities are conducted daily in every neonatal unit. We all practice pharmacovigilance, perhaps without knowing it. Explicit attention to pharmacovigilance will improve the quality of care given to individual babies as well as to the general population of neonates.

Table 1. Examples of adverse drug reactions in neonates that have influenced practice

Drug	ADR	Implication for practice
Chloral hydrate	Encephalopathy	Minimize use in extremely preterm neonates
Tolazoline	Oliguria, systemic hypotension	Develop new therapies (such as inhaled nitric oxide)
Indomethacin	Oliguria	Consider alternatives (such as ibuprofen)
Corticosteroids	Growth; brain development; hyperglycemia	Consider benefit-risk balance carefully
Vitamin E	Metabolic decompensation	Avoid formulations that have not been tested in neonates
Chloramphenicol	Grey-baby syndrome	Avoid formulations that have not been tested in neonates
Codeine	Respiratory depression	Be alert to age-specific pharmacogenetic effects
Oxygen	Retinopathy of prematurity at high doses. Death at low doses	Conduct appropriate clinical trials to define optimal thresholds
Sulfonamides	Kernicterus due to displacement of bilirubin from plasma proteins	Be alert to age-specific effects on distribution and age-specific effects of deranging physiology

One key element of avoiding medicine-related harm is avoiding errors. Errors arise when medicines are not used as intended, e.g., when a mistake with dilution leads to an overdose or to an underdose. In contrast, adverse drug reactions (ADRs) arise when medicines are used as intended. There is a significant amount of literature on medical errors in neonatal units [2]. We will not consider errors in this chapter. Harms can also arise from devices and from other interventions. Methods to detect and assess harms have broader relevance, but devices will not be considered here. Perinatal pharmacovigilance is also important. While it is important to detect the effects of drugs given to the mother before birth or during lactation, these topics are not included in this chapter. The aim of this chapter is to describe the assessment and mitigation of harms that arise directly from medicines that are used as intended in neonatal units.

Table 1 summarizes some ADRs that have influenced neonatal practice. The issues have been summarized with respect to the brain [3] and the kidney [4].

Pharmacovigilance in Clinical Practice

Real-time pharmacovigilance is essential to good neonatal care. ADRs often prompt adjustments to therapy.

First: Minimize risk by following good prescribing practice. This can be summarized as ensuring that the following are in place for every prescription:

- Clear indication
- Reasonable evidence base

- Reasonable benefit-risk balance
- Clear therapeutic objective for efficacy
- Ways to monitor whether the objective for efficacy is being met and to stop administering the medicine if it is not helping
- Clear markers of tolerable and intolerable adverse effects
- Ways to monitor whether adverse effects are present, supported by therapeutic drug monitoring if appropriate, and ways to stop administering the medicine if it is doing more harm than good
- Ways to reduce the exposure and to stop administering the medicine as soon as possible
- Performance of a review of known risk factors, such as renal impairment, both before prescribing and periodically during the course of administering the medicine.

At first, this section may appear to state the obvious. However, high-quality prescribing in neonates is difficult to implement and sustain when working across teams and in complex shift patterns. Pharmacy review can be extremely helpful. Teamwork and critical thinking are very useful. Unit guidelines provide the best basis for this work. Regular updates and prompts are needed to maintain awareness about this information.

Second: When a concern is raised, take a systematic approach [5]. Some steps may need to be compressed in an acute situation. It is well worth considering and documenting a systematic approach for addressing unexpected events. A systematic approach should include:

1. Clinical assessment of the adverse event
- Detailed history
- Focused physical diagnosis
- Focused investigations
- Analysis of drug exposure
- Review of all drug exposures

2. Differential diagnosis
- All possible clinical diagnoses considered

3. Review of predisposing factors
4. Review of the association between drug exposure and the adverse event
- Literature search (which may be local, comprising guidelines and formularies, or more extensive, comprising systematic literature reviews)
- Causality assessment (see below)

5. Management plan

The management plan needs to include three steps.

(a) Giving advice to professionals. This can include stopping the medication, changing the dose, changing the medication, mitigating the adverse effects, and performing follow-up.

(b) Communicating with families. Research about older children has found that parents often suspect that a child has suffered harm from a medicine and want to discuss this with professionals [6]. There is less available information about how parents view drug safety in neonatal units. There is clearly a balance between openness and excessive uncertainty, and skilled practitioners must make individualized judgments about specific families.

(c) Reporting to the institution, regulators and manufacturers. At the unit or institutional level, adverse drug reactions may prompt altered prescribing guidance. Many jurisdictions have databases for spontaneous reports of suspected adverse drug reactions. These can be powerful ways to detect and evaluate new adverse reactions. However, these databases depend on good reporting by clinicians. The manufacturers of medicines need to know about problems that arise with their products.

Generalizable Information about Drug Safety

This section is about approaches to pharmacovigilance that aim to gather robust information that is relevant to groups or populations of neonates.

Sharing Information about Drug Safety

The standard tools for pharmacovigilance include:

- Spontaneous reports of suspected ADRs to national or regional regulators. Important examples for neonates include Kaletra [7] and ceftriaxone [8].
- Published case reports. An important example in neonates is the relationship between codeine, respiratory suppression and the genetics of morphine metabolism [9].
- Clinical trials. Well-conducted clinical trials perform structured, prospective data collection. Control, or placebo, groups provide useful comparisons. The value of clinical trials is enhanced by paying attention to regulatory requirements — see below. Safety outcomes should be included in all neonatal clinical trials.
- Prospective observational studies. Cohort studies capture a group of participants, their exposure to medicines and the outcomes. These studies allow some control over some of the biases associated with observational studies [10].
- Retrospective observational studies. Case-control studies capture a group with an adverse outcome and examine how many of the people who experienced that adverse outcome were exposed to a particular medicine [10]. Case-control studies can be powerful, but they require good data collection systems in clinical practice to avoid biases from incomplete data.
- Prescription databases. These are used a great deal in other populations [10]. As electronic patient records and electronic prescribing increase, these sources of data could be used more with neonates. However, these approaches require careful attention to data entry and in general, electronic databases require careful attention to the definitions used for clinical conditions and outcomes. Clinical diagnoses may not be sufficient for adequate phenotyping.

- Surveillance. As noted above, spontaneous reporting can be a useful way to identify novel reports. Systematic attention to these reports by 'sentinel' units may add value to spontaneous reporting.

An important concept in pharmacovigilance is the 'signal'. A signal is an initial suspicion that requires further investigation. Some of the above-mentioned approaches to pharmacovigilance identify signals (case reports, surveillance), whereas others evaluate signals to a greater or lesser extent (cohort studies, case-control studies, clinical trials). It is often not possible to develop a conclusive estimate of whether a drug causes a particular ADR. Instead, well-designed studies can help clinicians to narrow the odds and to make informed decisions.

Population studies, including cohort studies, are popular in neonatology. One way to optimize cohort studies is to use a propensity score. These have been used to elucidate the relationships between pain and long-term outcomes, for example, by authors in The Netherlands [11]. Propensity scores aim to clarify the relationship between exposures (such as exposure to medicines) and adverse outcomes by adjusting for the risk of the adverse outcome before the exposure.

Causality

A key issue in pharmacovigilance is determining whether a medicine has contributed to the causation of an event. Causality can be assessed in a variety of ways, including performing a comprehensive review of information and making a decision about causality based on 'global introspection'. Checklists, algorithms and scoring systems such as the Naranjo score can be used. This scoring system has limitations, but it has been modified for use in neonates [12]. An alternative is to use specific criteria to make the judgment: a criterion-based assessment tool has been validated in children [13].

Severity and Avoidability

The impact of a drug-related ADR is important. There is a difference between 'severity', which has a specific regulatory meaning (see Section 'Pharmacovigilance in Clinical Trials'), and 'seriousness', which is the perception of impact by clinicians or families. This issue is complicated because the extent to which a drug can be blamed for an adverse event is often unclear. In practice, a root cause analysis or similar approach may be needed. In research settings, it is important to use one of the commonly used tools consistently, notwithstanding imperfections in the published tools.

Classifying ADRs

People have classified pharmacologic and idiosyncratic ADRs with varying levels of sophistication [14]. The distinctions have broken down as knowledge about pharmacology has expanded, and it has become clear that many agents have many targets. Immunologically mediated ADRs appear to be very rare in neonates, presumably because of the age-specific pattern of immune activity.

Pharmacogenetics

Genes can affect how an individual responds to medicines, modifying the chances of successful treatment and increasing the risks of adverse drug reactions. It is important that clinicians and researchers be alert to the possibility that genetic effects may be important causes of unexplained symptoms [9]. Pharmacogenetics are relevant to many medicines given to neonates, although neonatal pharmacogenetics is a young science [15].

Specific Features of Pharmacovigilance in the NICU

A number of features of babies and the care they receive are relevant to clinical and generalizable pharmacovigilance in the NICU.

Intensive care in any age group hinders pharmacovigilance. Sick neonates may have many conditions, making it difficult to distinguish between the harms that arise from treatments and those that are consequences of underlying conditions. One aspect of this situation is 'confounding by indication'. Medicines are used to treat conditions. Problems that arise after starting to administer the medicine may be due to the underlying condition or due to the medicine. The only way to definitively overcome confounding by indication is through randomized trials. However, performing trials for safety effects may be difficult to justify, thus reinforcing the need to capture safety data reliably during trials for efficacy.

Sick neonates are treated with multiple medicines. It is difficult to identify which medicines cause harm. The pattern of medicines used to treat neonates has changed with time, as has the pattern of ADRs observed in neonates.

Some specific characteristics of neonates complicate pharmacovigilance. As described 30–40 years ago, sick neonates have a number of risk factors for ADRs. These include extreme prematurity, complications of prematurity (respiratory distress syndrome, intraventricular hemorrhage, necrotizing enterocolitis, apnea), illness severity (elevated hepatic transaminases, renal failure) and treatments (ventilation, parenteral nutrition) [16]. The underlying conditions and organ immaturity observed in neonates manifest with physiological instability, leading to a high incidence of background events which are not necessarily an indication of drug-related harm or of clinical deterioration. Examples include episodes of bradycardia and desaturation.

Ontogeny affects the handling of drugs (pharmacokinetics, PK) and their effects (PD). Age-specific features of PK that can affect the likelihood of ADRs in neonates include the extent of drug bioavailability due to differences in gastric acidity or gastric emptying, the pattern of distribution due to altered proportions of body water and fat, age-specific patterns of metabolism (although these are generally poorly described) and the extent of elimination. Renal elimination in neonates is less than that in older age groups because of reduced glomerular filtration and because of differences in the expression of tubular proteins (summarized in other chapters of this book).

Ontogeny includes unique stages, and effects may therefore be limited to specific points in development. Furthermore, there can be significant delays before adverse effects become apparent. Adverse effects can disrupt processes that affect later aspects of development.

The possibility of adverse reactions may be raised in other settings. For example, many xenobiotics will cause adverse findings in cellular models, animals or adults. Often, these effects occur at much higher exposures than those observed in neonates. The relevance of findings from in vitro or in vivo studies is often unclear. These theoretical possibilities may reduce the willingness of clinicians to use helpful medicines.

The long-term effects of administering medication to neonates are not well understood. This should be reflected in the arrangements for long-term follow-up.

In the future, drug development will involve fewer patients than it has before. In general, regulators try to reduce barriers by streamlining studies that put medicines on the market, leading, in some cases, to a focus on efficacy for the primary marketing authorization. A more sophisticated approach to safety assessment during drug development [17] and a need to gather safety data in post-marketing studies [18] will be needed. This is particularly true for neonates, as there is an ethical requirement to minimize the number of neonates recruited to clinical trials. There are also relatively few neonates in the context of the large numbers of indications for medicines in this population. These constraints are being overcome though creative work that makes the best use of the existing information when designing clinical trials for neonates. Work involving extrapolation and modeling will lead to useful results from tests performed on relatively small numbers of babies (Chapter 7, this volume, pp 83–107). These approaches often assume that a medicine works in the same way in different age groups so that its efficacy can be extrapolated. If that assumption holds, then trials for efficacy will not be performed. In many indications, a marketing authorization for neonates depends on studies that indicate the doses that are needed. While safety assessments are included in these studies, they do not include enough participants to give a comprehensive view of the safety of the medication. Thus, in neonates, there is an even greater need to continue post-marketing surveillance to ensure that drug labels based on extrapolated data have an appropriate benefit-risk balance.

Pharmacovigilance in Clinical Trials

This section refers to pharmacovigilance during clinical trials of investigational medicinal products (fig. 1). These interventional studies provide a unique opportunity to study safety. Clinical trials are used to determine treatment for many future babies. When drawing conclusions from trials, information about harms needs to be balanced against information about benefits. Therefore, it is important to gather data about adverse events systematically. There are legal and ethical requirements for pharmacovigilance. All clinicians caring for neonates enrolled in trials have a duty to report

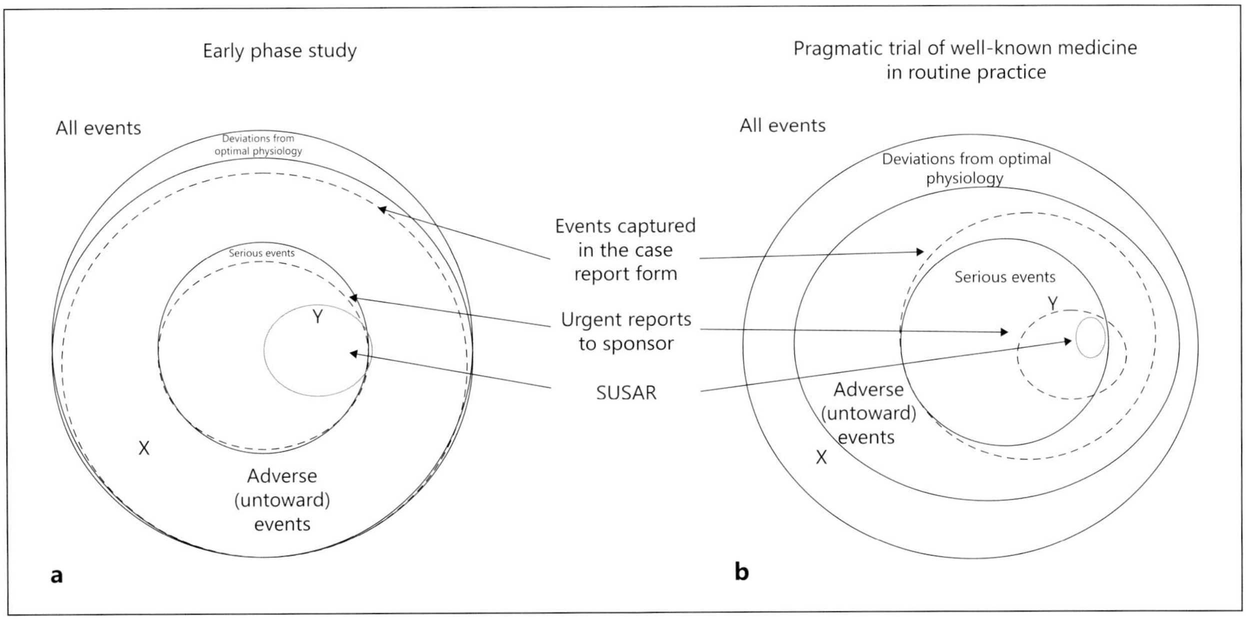

Fig. 1. Different types of events and how they can relate to reporting. This figure demonstrates how clinical events relate to the classification of events used in the regulatory assessment of pharmacovigilance. The solid circles indicate different types of events (with labels in the figure). The dashed circles indicate different approaches to reporting (with labels between the figures). In neonates, frequent deviations from optimal physiology may not be adverse events, or the sponsor may not wish to record them in the CRF. When a novel drug is tested, the sponsor will be thorough about describing what should be recorded and what should be reported urgently (**a**). Most of the events will be captured in the CRF, and many events may be reported urgently to the sponsor. When a drug is well-known and is being used according to routine clinical practice, the sponsor can be selective about what is reported urgently (**b**). In a study of a well-known medicine, fewer events are captured in the CRF, and there are fewer urgent reports to the sponsor. Event X may be recorded in the CRF in an early-phase study. The event may turn out to be common and may not be relevant to the safety assessment of the medicine. In that case, it may not be recorded in the CRF in a pragmatic trial. Serious event Y may be unexpected in an early-phase study and may lead to a SUSAR report. In the pragmatic trial, it may be recognized as a serious event observed during treatment and may not need urgent reporting to the sponsor.

events that contribute to safety assessments. It is therefore essential for all clinicians to understand how safety is studied in clinical trials. Neonates have different profiles of adverse events of background diseases. Using the safety sections from protocols defined for other populations is not appropriate. Accordingly, neonatologists need to advise sponsors about the safety issues in clinical trial protocols. This account draws on experiences in the UK, but the principles are similar in other jurisdictions [19].

It is important to recognize that the language used to describe adverse events in clinical trials is different from the language used to describe adverse events in clinical practice. Some events may need to be urgently reviewed by the agencies that regulate drugs because new information about a study medicine may be relevant to future participants in the trial or may need to be widely disseminated. This means that the sponsors of clinical trials have a responsibility to report some events to regulatory agencies urgently in what is called 'expedited reporting'. Accordingly, investigators need to report some events urgently to the sponsor of a trial. The actions required of sponsors and investigators depend on what is known about the drug. There are specific terms that are used to describe adverse events during clinical trials. These terms indicate how the events are handled during the trial and which events require urgent reporting to the regulators.

The sponsor decides which non-serious adverse events need to be recorded in the trial record, the case report form (CRF) that is completed for each participant in a clinical trial. The choice about which adverse events are recorded in the CRF is based on the aims of the study. Studies of well-known or widely used drugs are likely to collect less, more focused, safety information than studies of drugs that have not been previously used in neonates. Given the lack of information about drug safety in neonates, it is often advisable to collect systematic data about known safety events to refine estimates of the frequency of adverse events in neonates. Sick neonates have many derangements in physiology. Some of these derangements are common and have no effect on the trial outcome; examples include desaturation and bradycardia. Accordingly, the sponsor can elect not to include them in the protocol. If the investigator believes that an event that is usually not harmful is so severe that it is causing harm, then that event should be recorded in the CRF, and other action should be considered. The protocol can require urgent reporting of non-serious adverse events if the events are critical for the evaluation of safety in the trial.

Clinicians frequently assess and describe how sick a baby is. During a clinical trial, the severity of illness is different from the seriousness of an event. There is a specific regulatory definition of 'seriousness' (table 2); this is intended to promote the consistent reporting of events that need to be assessed urgently by drug regulators.

Adverse events need to be assessed for whether they are related to the study intervention (causality) and for whether they are expected to occur with that drug in that population. There are many ways to assess causality. Investigators need to become familiar with whichever causality assessment the sponsor has chosen. The key distinction is made between events that are unlikely to have been caused by a study drug and those that are possibly due to the study drug (or where causality is more likely than it is possible).

During a clinical trial, an adverse reaction is expected if it appears on a trial-related document known as the reference safety information (RSI). The RSI can appear in the protocol, on the drug label (in Europe, the summary of product characteristics) or in the document used to inform the investigator about the drug if it is not licensed (the investigator's brochure). Anticipated reactions are only expected from a regulatory perspective if the events appear in the RSI. These events can be included in the RSI. Sponsors need to take advice from neonatologists about what goes into the RSI for

Table 2. Definitions of terms used during pharmacovigilance in clinical trials

Term	Definition
Adverse event	An event that occurs during the administration of a medicine and that may or may not be related to the medicine. Sponsors can select which adverse events are related in the case report form.
Serious adverse event	An adverse event that is one of the following: death; life-threatening illness; permanent disability; congenital anomaly; requires hospitalization or an extended hospital stay. All serious adverse events must be recorded in the case report form.
Important event	An event that requires medical intervention to prevent a serious adverse event. Many sponsors view important events as being similar to serious adverse events.
Adverse reaction	An event that is related to a drug. There are several ways to determine whether an event is related to a drug. An event is unrelated if it can be explained by underlying illnesses or if there is no reason to link the drug to the event.
Serious adverse reaction	An event that is related to a drug and that involves an event included in the definition of a serious adverse event.
Expected event	An event that is included in the reference safety information, such as in the summary of product characteristics or in specific sections of the protocol.
Suspected unexpected serious adverse reaction (SUSAR)	An event that is not listed in the reference safety information that is related to a drug and that fulfils one of the criteria for a serious event. SUSARs must be reported to the regulators and to the ethics committee in strict timetables (expedited reports). This means that investigators must report potential SUSARs to the sponsor urgently, usually within 24 hours. Reporting potential SUSARs to the sponsor involves a significant amount of time and effort. Unless there is a thorough list of expected events in a neonatal protocol, many events will be unexpected and will require urgent reporting to the sponsor. A key part of designing neonatal clinical trials is designing the safety aspects of the protocol so that true SUSARs are reported urgently and that nuisance reporting is minimized.
Sponsor	The organization with responsibility for the quality assurance of all aspects of a trial. This includes deciding which aspects of safety are recorded in the case report form and ensuring that the regulators and the ethics committees are promptly informed of SUSARs.
Intercurrent event	An event that is part of the underlying illness and that is not related to the trial intervention. For example, in a trial of progesterone during early pregnancy, maternal hospitalization after delivery to treat an infected episiotomy would be an intercurrent event.

neonatal trials. Because the drug label, or the summary of product characteristics, does not usually focus on neonates, the RSI needs to be included in the protocol (or in the investigator's brochure).

The events that require urgent reporting to the regulators are those that are serious (see definition in table 2), those that are possibly caused by the drug (or more likely than not to be caused) and those that do not appear on the RSI. These are suspected, unexpected serious adverse reactions (SUSARs). It is important to report SUSARs that need urgent assessment. It is useful to avoid reporting events that do not need urgent assessment.

Neonates have many serious adverse events that are 'anticipated' as part of the underlying illness, including death. Clinicians may see these events frequently in clinical practice, and the events may be defined in the protocol as anticipated. They may then be exempt from expedited reporting to the regulators.

In order to meet their duties to report SUSARs urgently, sponsors need to know about serious adverse reactions urgently; this means that investigators are required to report serious adverse reactions to the sponsor urgently. Serious adverse reactions are common in sick neonates. The sponsor may not want to know about expected serious adverse reactions and can list the serious adverse reactions it does not want urgent notification of in the RSI. The events are still reported non-urgently and are evaluated to determine whether their incidence is greater than the anticipated incidence, in which case they are reported as SUSARs.

When drugs are first used in neonates, the sponsor is likely to want to assess safety more closely than when a drug has been used for some time. It is important to identify key safety events while avoiding nuisance reporting; this requires careful planning of trials in neonates.

Even if events are not reported urgently, it is important to capture them for meta-analysis across multiple trials.

Excipients Can Cause Adverse Reactions

The roles of excipients in medicines given to neonates are described elsewhere in this volume. Neonates are exposed to significant amounts of excipients [20]. Prototypical examples of safety issues are related to propylene glycol. The natural history of adverse events associated with propylene glycol has been described. The presence or absence of these events in routine clinical practice can be detected from the results of natural experiments arising from the use of different drug formulations [21]. These natural experiments have been supplemented by excipient kinetic studies. At the concentrations administered to most neonates, the exposure is unlikely to cause short-term effects to these patients. However, long-term toxicity cannot be ruled out. The situation may be different if propylene glycol is co-administered with ethanol, as indicated by the experience with Kaletra [7].

Excipients in plastics and medical devices may also lead to safety concerns. These excipients include bisphenol A (BPA) and phthalates [22].

The assessment of safety issues arising from excipients needs to account for the reasons why excipients are included in medicines. It may not be possible to supply a stable or sterile dosage form if excipients are avoided. Although it may be difficult to exclude the possibility of long-term adverse effects, it will be helpful to consider the concentrations required to cause cellular effects that could cause underlying outcomes. Measurements of circulating exposures will then allow an estimate of whether an appropriate safety margin can be applied.

Conclusions

In clinical practice, it is important to consider ADRs as a possible cause of unexplained symptoms. Notably, 5% of hospital admissions among adults are due to an ADR [23], and 15% of adults experience an ADR during admission [24]; 3% of hospital admissions among children involve an ADR [25]. Neonates have a number of risk factors for ADRs, which means that ADRs are likely to complicate neonatal care. When addressing a new clinical problem, it is important to ask whether this problem is related to a drug and whether a change to a medicine is likely to reduce the impact of the problem.

Good pharmacovigilance is a combination of individual surveillance and good systems. Good systems do not happen by accident and need constant attention and support.

Clinical trials are an ideal setting in which to describe the nature and frequency of ADRs. All staff in neonatal units that conduct clinical trials should be aware of the need to report adverse events in a way that meets regulatory requirements.

Research into pharmacovigilance is exciting and is likely to yield direct patient benefits. Good research requires a good study design and careful capturing of clinical data.

References

1 World Health Organization: Pharmacovigilance. [cited 2012 23rd March]; Available from: http://www.who.int/medicines/areas/quality_safety/safety_efficacy/pharmvigi/en/index.html.

2 Chedoe I, Molendijk HA, Dittrich ST, Jansman FG, Harting JW, Brouwers JR, et al: Incidence and nature of medication errors in neonatal intensive care with strategies to improve safety: a review of the current literature. Drug Saf 2007;30:503–513.

3 Gressens P, Rogido M, Paindaveine B, Sola A: The impact of neonatal intensive care practices on the developing brain. J Pediatr 2002;140:646–653.

4 Zaffanello M, Bassareo PP, Cataldi L, Antonucci R, Biban P, Fanos V: Long-term effects of neonatal drugs on the kidney. J Matern Fetal Neonatal Med 2010;23(suppl 3):87–89.

5 Rieder MJ: In vivo and in vitro testing for adverse drug reactions. Pediatr Clin North Am 1997;44:93–111.

6 Arnott J, Hesselgreaves H, Nunn AJ, Peak M, Pirmohamed M, Smyth RL, et al: Enhancing communication about paediatric medicines: lessons from a qualitative study of parents' experiences of their child's suspected adverse drug reaction. PloS One 2012;7:e46022.

7 U.S. Food and Drug Administration: FDA Drug Safety Communication: Serious health problems seen in premature babies given Kaletra (lopinavir/ritonavir) oral solution. 2011 [cited]; Available from: http://www.fda.gov/Drugs/DrugSafety/ucm246002.htm.

8 Bradley JS, Wassel RT, Lee L, Nambiar S: Intravenous ceftriaxone and calcium in the neonate: assessing the risk for cardiopulmonary adverse events. Pediatrics 2009;123:e609–e613.

9 Koren G, Cairns J, Chitayat D, Gaedigk A, Leeder SJ: Pharmacogenetics of morphine poisoning in a breastfed neonate of a codeine-prescribed mother. Lancet 2006;368:704.

10 Strom BL, Kimmel SE, Hennessy S: Textbook of Pharmacoepidemiology, ed 2. Chichester, West Sussex, John Wiley & Sons, 2013.

11 de Graaf J, van Lingen RA, Valkenburg AJ, Weisglas-Kuperus N, Groot Jebbink L, Wijnberg-Williams B, et al: Does neonatal morphine use affect neuropsychological outcomes at 8 to 9 years of age? Pain 2013;154:449–458.

12 Du W, Lehr VT, Lieh-Lai M, Koo W, Ward RM, Rieder MJ, et al: An algorithm to detect adverse drug reactions in the neonatal intensive care unit. J Clin Pharmacol 2013;53:87–95.

13 Gallagher RM, Kirkham JJ, Mason JR, Bird KA, Williamson PR, Nunn AJ, et al: Development and inter-rater reliability of the Liverpool adverse drug reaction causality assessment tool. PloS One 2011;6:e28096.
14 Edwards IR, Aronson JK: Adverse drug reactions: definitions, diagnosis, and management. Lancet 2000;356:1255–1259.
15 Allegaert K: Mechanism based medicine in infancy: complex interplay between developmental pharmacology and pharmacogenetics. Int J Clin Pharm 2011;33:473–474.
16 Knight M: Adverse drug reactions in neonates. J Clin Pharmacol 1994;34:128–135.
17 Ray A: Beyond debacle and debate: developing solutions in drug safety. Nat Rev Drug Discov 2009;8:775–779.
18 Callreus T: The new EU legislation on pharmacovigilance and changing models for drug development. Drug Saf 2011;34:529–530; author reply 530–531.
19 Medicines and Healthcare Products Regulatory Agency: Good Clinical Practice Guide. London, The Stationery Office, 2012.
20 Lass J, Naelapaa K, Shah U, Kaar R, Varendi H, Turner MA, et al: Hospitalised neonates in Estonia commonly receive potentially harmful excipients. BMC Pediatr 2012;12:136.
21 Allegaert K, Vanhaesebrouck S, Kulo A, Cosaert K, Verbesselt R, Debeer A, et al: Prospective assessment of short-term propylene glycol tolerance in neonates. Arch Dis Child 2010;95:1054–1058.
22 Pak VM, Nailon RE, McCauley LA: Controversy: neonatal exposure to plasticizers in the NICU. MCN Am J Matern Child Nurs 2007;32:244–249.
23 Pirmohamed M, James S, Meakin S, Green C, Scott AK, Walley TJ, et al: Adverse drug reactions as cause of admission to hospital: prospective analysis of 18,820 patients. BMJ 2004;329:15–19.
24 Davies EC, Green CF, Taylor S, Williamson PR, Mottram DR, Pirmohamed M: Adverse drug reactions in hospital in-patients: a prospective analysis of 3,695 patient-episodes. PloS One 2009;4:e4439.
25 Gallagher RM, Mason JR, Bird KA, Kirkham JJ, Peak M, Williamson PR, et al: Adverse drug reactions causing admission to a paediatric hospital. PloS One 2012;7:e50127.

Dr. Mark Turner
Neonatal Unit, Liverpool Women's Hospital
Crown Street
Liverpool L8 7SS (UK)
E-Mail mark.turner@liverpool.ac.uk

Mimouni FB, van den Anker JN (eds): Neonatal Pharmacology and Nutrition Update.
Pediatr Adolesc Med. Basel, Karger, 2015, vol 18, pp 41–57 (DOI: 10.1159/000365021)

Neonatal Formulations and Additives

Karel Allegaert[a] · Mark A. Turner[b] · Johannes N. van den Anker[c–f]

[a]Neonatal Intensive Care Unit, University Hospitals Leuven, Leuven, Belgium; [b]Department of Women's and Children's Health, Institute of Translational Medicine, University of Liverpool, Liverpool, UK; [c]Division of Pediatric Clinical Pharmacology, Children's National Medical Center, Washington, DC, and [d]Departments of Pediatrics, Pharmacology, Physiology and Integrative Systems Biology, George Washington University School of Medicine and Health Sciences, Washington DC, USA; [e]Intensive Care, Erasmus MC- Sophia Children's Hospital, Rotterdam, The Netherlands; [f]Department of Paediatric Pharmacology, University Children's Hospital, Basel, Switzerland

Abstract

Neonatal drug dosing needs to be based on the physiological characteristics of the newborn and pharmacokinetic parameters of the drug. Overall, clearance is lower in neonates when compared to children or adults. In addition, there is already extensive between-individual variability in clearance in the first months of life. As a consequence, there is a need for an appropriate balance between dose, volume, drug manipulations and dose flexibility in neonates that calls for dedicated and tailored formulations. During the development of these formulations, there is also a need to quantify and limit excipient exposure based on the currently available knowledge on their safety and toxicity. Furthermore, focused studies on the clinical pharmacology of excipients in neonates should be conducted. Finally, until tailored vials and formulations become available, compounding practices for drug formulations in neonates should be evaluated to guarantee correct dosing, product stability and safety.

Introduction: The Need for Tailored Formulations in Neonates

Neonatal drug dosing needs to be based on both the physiological characteristics of the newborn and the pharmacokinetic parameters of the drug [1–3]. Overall, drug clearance is lower in neonates when compared to children or adults. However, size-related changes can only, in part, be modelled based on allometry and can be associated with the observation that the metabolic rate relates to weight by a $kg^{0.75}$ trend. Indeed, in addition to size, other population-specific covariates (e.g. co-medication, asphyxia, growth restriction, postnatal age, postmenstrual age) further contribute to

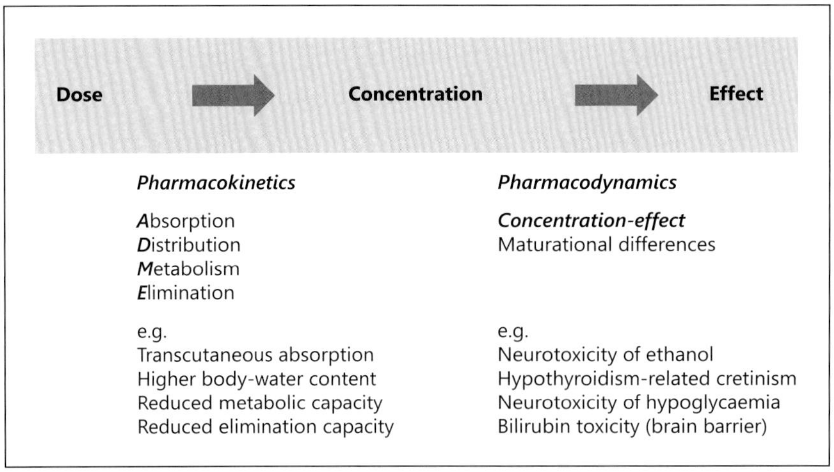

Fig. 1. Pharmacokinetics and pharmacodynamics in neonates.

the inter-individual variability in clearance within a neonatal population [4, 5]. However, the limited size (0.5–5 kg) does not preclude an extensive, i.e. commonly at least a 10-fold, variability in clearance within this specific group of patients. Population-specific pharmacodynamics *(concentration-effect profile)* can only be evaluated after population-specific pharmacokinetics *(concentration-time profile)* have been considered (fig. 1) [1–7]. For a more extensive review on the issues of developmental pharmacokinetics and the integration of pharmacokinetics and pharmacodynamics, we refer to Chapters 3 and 4 of this book.

The combination of an overall low clearance with extensive variability within the neonatal age ranges results in the need for low and adjustable dosing in early life [5, 6]. As a consequence, when tailoring formulations for neonates, these prerequisites, i.e. low, flexible dosing of a given drug, need to be considered [7]. Because of specific disease characteristics, the commonly used methods for administering formulations include vials for intravenous administration, oral drops or liquids (e.g. suspension, syrup). In addition to the parent compounds, these formulations contain excipients, which are needed as co-solvents, surfactants (a general term for compounds that improve absorption; it is unrelated to the lung surfactant that is administered for hyaline membrane disease), preservatives, colorants and/or sweeteners [8–11].

However, the above-mentioned, maturational pharmacokinetics and pharmacodynamics are not limited to only the active compounds but are also relevant for excipients and additives that are co-administered as part of a specific formulation [8, 9]. Examples of such excipients are lactose, aspartame, ethanol, propylene glycol, benzyl alcohol, sorbitol, xylitol, mannitol and poly-ethylene glycol. Besides their disease-specific aspects (e.g. lactose in the setting of lactase deficiency, aspartame in the setting of patients suffering from phenylketonuria, or fructose-containing formulations in the setting of fructose intolerance), nearly all medicines are formulated with excipients that have been used for many years and are Generally Regarded As Safe, which is reflected in the 'GRAS' status [11–14]. However, this 'GRAS' status does not consider the population-specific pharmacokinetics and pharmacodynamics of neonates [6, 7, 14]. Similarly, these claims are not always based on well-validated prospective studies in neonates [12, 13, 15]. Another example to support this finding is the fact that exposure to sorbitol or xylitol potentially results in diarrhoea and even metabolic hyperchloraemic acidosis [16].

Those Who Cannot Remember the Past are Condemned to Repeat It (G. Sabtatana)
History provides us with illustrations on the relevance of excipient-related toxicity in newborns [5, 12, 17]. Benzyl alcohol, propylene glycol, thimerosal and ethanol will be used as illustrations of the relevance of excipients for drug development in neonates.

Fatal benzyl alcohol-related poisoning has been described in a case series of low-birth-weight (<1,500 g, n = 10) infants after co-administration of this excipient as a bacteriostatic agent for normal saline administration [18–21]. Following exposure to at least 130 mg/kg of benzyl alcohol, these neonates developed metabolic acidosis and had an elevated Anion Gap from the second day of exposure onwards with subsequent development of a clinical picture that included progressive bradycardia, gasping and seizures [18–21]. Following this event, evidence emerged that this clinical syndrome in neonates was related to maturational deficiency of the benzyl alcohol degradation (benzyl alcohol to benzoic acid to hippuric acid) capacity [18–21].

Similarly, the toxicity of propylene glycol in preterm neonates (<1,500 g) has also been documented [22–27]. Preterm neonates developed biochemical abnormalities (e.g. hyperosmolarity, lactic acidosis, elevated creatinine and bilirubin concentrations) following exposure to up to 3,000 mg/day of propylene glycol for at least 5 consecutive days. These biochemical abnormalities resulted in clinical symptoms, including seizures and bradycardic episodes [22–27].

Although both case observations took place in the early 1980s, the issue of propylene glycol toxicity is still relevant today. In 2011, the Food and Drug Administration (FDA) notified healthcare professionals of the relevant health problems reported in preterm neonates exposed to Kaletra® (lopinavir/ritonavir) oral solution [28]. Kaletra® is an antiviral drug commonly used in combination with other antiretroviral drugs for the treatment of Human Immunodeficiency Virus (HIV). Kaletra® contained both propylene glycol (152.7 mg/5 ml) and ethanol (42% v/v). The association between Kaletra® exposure and cardiac, renal and respiratory symptoms in early neonatal life was described and resulted in the suggestion to avoid this formulation in (pre)term neonates until the postmenstrual age of 42 weeks was reached.

The discussion on the safety of thimerosal-containing vaccines (TCVs) started in 1999 with a joint statement issued by the American Academy of Pediatrics and the U.S. Public Health Service calling for measures to remove thimerosal from vaccines used in infants [29–33]. This resulted in the absence of TCVs routinely used in the

United States and the European Union to protect preschool children (Center of Disease Control, 2004, European Medicines Agency, 2001). This decision was mainly based on in vitro and animal experimental observations on the neurotoxicity of the mercury present in thimerosal. However, some countries continue to use TCVs in childhood immunization schedules. The World Health Organisation's (WHO) position is based on the high effectiveness of vaccines in protecting children against infectious diseases and not on specific studies addressing ethyl mercury in population studies [29–33]. A recent prospective, neurodevelopmental follow-up cohort study in 196 neonates in the region of Krakow showed that there was no clinical evidence for developmental delays associated with TCV exposure in the first 3 years of life [34]. However, the authors explicitly referred to the risk of subtle negative influences on psychomotor development when neonates at birth were exposed to TCVs because the mercury levels in serum were not only higher but remained higher for a longer period, likely due to the reduced clearance capacity in neonates [34]. These recent observations confirmed the overall conclusions of Thompson et al. [32]. Among 42 neuropsychological outcomes that were assessed in 1,047 children, only a few significant associations with exposure to mercury from thimerosal were found [32]. Moreover, these associations were small and almost equally divided between positive and negative effects. Higher prenatal mercury exposure was associated with better performance on one measure of language and with poorer performance on one measure of attention and executive functioning. Increasing levels of mercury exposure from birth to 7 months were associated with better performance on one measure of fine motor coordination and on one measure of attention and executive functioning. Increasing mercury exposure from birth to 28 days was associated with poorer performance on one measure of speech articulation and with better performance on one measure of fine motor coordination [32]. As a consequence, the authors of this report and other investigators concluded that there was no causal association between early exposure to mercury from TCVs and thimerosal-containing immune globulins and deficits in neuropsychological functioning at the age of 7–10 years [29–34]. To a certain extent, the same rationale can be considered for aluminium-containing formulations for immunization, which illustrates the difficult balance between the documentation of side effects compared to that of the absence of side effects [33].

Maturational pharmacodynamics should be considered in addition to maturational pharmacokinetics. Ethanol is known to be a neurotoxic compound with an age-specific impact on the fetal or neonatal brain (i.e. apoptosis and impaired synaptogenesis) with e.g. fetal alcohol syndrome [35]. We hereby have to be aware that, in preterm neonates, brain growth and maturation during the 3rd trimester is mainly an extra-uterine event.

Improved understanding of both pharmacokinetic and pharmacodynamic observations is needed to avoid the tragic events associated with early exposure to benzyl alcohol, propylene glycol, thimerosal, or ethanol [17–35]. Moreover, quantification of

Table 1. An overview of the kind of excipients commonly used for systemic exposure to each formulation

Formulation	Co-solvents	Surfactants	Preservatives	Colorants	Sweeteners
Intravenous	+	+	sometimes	–	–
Intramuscular	+	+	–	–	–
Oral liquid	+	+	+	not recommended	+
Tablets/capsules	–	+	–	not recommended	+

In neonates, intravenous formulations and oral liquid (syrup, suspension or drops) are most commonly used.

the lower thresholds of excipient-specific safety is needed to enable further tailored product development [7, 12, 23, 36].

Aspects of excipient use in any drug formulation will be discussed first (2), and this will subsequently be applied to the population of interest, i.e. preterm and term newborns (3). Tailored formulations that result in accurate dosing in neonates are obviously not limited to only excipient tailoring, and a roadmap for further improvements related to formulations for use in neonates has been suggested (4). We hereby will consider issues related to the relevance of dose accuracy, retrieval of already available information, and the need and feasibility for additional, focused studies on drug formulations in neonates in order to generate valid data on drug safety in neonates.

Excipients in Drug Formulations: Compounds Routinely Administered but Never Prescribed

Besides the active compound(s), drug formulations contain solvents and additives, which are usually referred to as 'excipients'. The United States' National Formulary uses a more dynamic definition of excipient: 'everything in the formulation in addition to the active compound(s)'. Excipient refers to any substance that is used as a vehicle or additive for administering drugs at a suitable consistency or in a suitable formulation [37–41]. These excipients are added, for example, to ensure stability over a given shelf life, to improve palatability, to facilitate solubility or to bulk up formulations that otherwise contain highly potent active ingredients, and these excipients are referred to as preservatives, sweeteners, fillers, solvents, coating materials or colouring agents. Table 1 provides a summary of the type of excipients commonly used per form of dosage [37–41]. As mentioned earlier, intravenous formulations and oral liquids are the preferred dosage forms for neonates [42].

Excipients have long been considered to be pharmacologically inactive but, in fact, they might cause adverse effects. It has to be kept in mind, particularly when excipients are used in paediatric formulations, that newborn physiology differs considerably from that of children or adults and even differs within the neonatal population [1, 4, 5, 7]. Maturational clearance processes may limit the elimination capacity and result in accumulation-related side effects [3, 23]. Likewise, maturational differences in pharmacodynamics (e.g. ethanol effects in the newborn) may result in age-specific side effects [35]. Moreover, pharmaceutical excipients are not always 'innocent' bystanders [41]. The small intestinal transit time, but not the gastric emptying time, of small, non-disintegrating tablets is affected by the iso-osmotic pharmaceutical excipient solution [43]. The gastric emptying time is shorter when a paracetamol formulation is alkalic ('effervescent tablet'), resulting in faster duodenal absorption and the subsequent effects. Transcutaneous absorption, in part, depends on the lipophilic characteristics of the formulation. For aerosolized formulations, the extent of pulmonary disposition, in part, depends on the size of the generated particles.

Similarly, liposomal amphotericin results in improved renal tubule tolerance because the structure of the liposome causes reduced reabsorption at the level of the renal tubule-cell brush border [44]. The amphotericin example already refers to the concept of 'functionality'. As recently reviewed by Hamman and Steenekamp, the concept of 'functionality' has been introduced by adding excipients to enhance product performance, e.g. membrane permeability, solubility, preventing degradation, controlling drug release or facilitating manufacturing [41]. Excipients are not always just innocent bystanders of a given formulation.

Limited permeability across biological membranes (e.g. the intestinal barrier, the blood-brain barrier) is one of the most significant obstacles to prevent achievement of therapeutic levels in the effected compartment. The bio-availability of Kaletra (lopinavir/ritonavir) is facilitated by adding Cremophor EL, which acts as a surfactant, to the formulation [45]. Animal experimental work suggests that erythropoietin (EPO) may serve as a neuroprotective agent in preterm neonates and term neonates with perinatal asphyxia. Recently, it has been documented that the transfer of a nano-formulation (human recombinant EPO, PLGA-EPO nanoparticles) through the blood-brain barrier results in a 10-fold higher bio-availability of the nano-formulation in the compartment of interest, i.e. the central nervous system [46]. Similarly, the efficacy of inactivated influenza vaccines is known to be poor in infants, but the use of an oil-in-water emulsion adjuvant results in more effective protection, which is defined by a reduction in influenza-attack rates [47].

Based on both the specific characteristics of the newborn and the 'functionality' concept of the excipients, the suitability of a specific excipient in a neonatal formulation is a crucial element of the pharmaceutical development process for new compounds, and the currently administered formulations need persistent consideration [9, 36]. This also means that, during the product-development process, a switch from an initially studied preliminary formulation to a commercial formulation should be supported by relevant bridging studies between different formulations that include bioequivalent studies in the population of interest [48].

Table 2. Commonly reported population-specific side effects of excipient exposure in neonates

Specific side effect	Excipient
Raised hyperbilirubinaemia	Parabens (methyl and propyl parahydroxybenzoate) sodium benzoate
Seizures	propylene glycol accumulation benzyl alcohol accumulation
Central nervous system depression	ethanol accumulation propylene glycol accumulation
Liver dysfunction, cholestasis	propylene glycol accumulation polysorbate 80
Metabolic acidosis	propylene glycol accumulation polysorbate 80 benzyl alcohol

Excipients for Formulations in Newborns

Although the above-mentioned case observations on benzyl alcohol, propylene glycol or thimerosal reflect the potential impact of inappropriate exposure of neonates to excipients, we should be aware that exposure of neonates to excipients is common in our neonatal intensive care environment, irrespective of the formulations used [12, 49]. In general, the selection of an excipient for neonatal formulations should consider its pharmaceutical form (e.g. vials, drops, liquids), the available data on its safety profile in neonates, the expected duration of treatment (e.g. single, short or long term), and the potential for allergies and sensitization [8, 9, 48]. Finally, novel excipients with no paediatric safety information should be avoided, and consequently, excipients with an established track record are preferred [48]. Some clinical toxicological syndromes in neonates that are linked with specific excipients are provided in table 2.

Whittaker et al. recently reported both the incidence and the extent of exposure to some of the more commonly administered excipients in oral formulations in one neonatal intensive care unit [12]. The authors described that the eligible target group (birth weight <1,500 g, n = 38) was exposed to at least 20 different excipients, including *'assumed to be toxic excipients'* like ethanol or propylene glycol. To further illustrate this, liquid formulations with furosemide or dexamethasone, which are commonly administered to neonates with bronchopulmonary dysplasia, resulted in significant exposure to ethanol [12]. Significant exposure was defined as at least 1 ethanol unit/week for an adult man. Similarly, some infants were exposed to sorbitol, even at levels in excess of the recommended guidelines for the maximal daily exposure (/kg) in adults. Finally, co-administration of propylene glycol with a dexamethasone liquid formulation commonly resulted in a weekly exposure above the 150-mg/kg/week limit for adults [12].

Shehab et al. quantified both benzyl alcohol and propylene glycol exposures in a cohort of critically ill neonates and young infants [22]. Based on 170 episodes of either benzyl alcohol (n = 88) or propylene glycol (n = 82) exposure in such infants, a wide range in cumulative excipient dose was documented, with a median cumulative dose of 4.5 mg/kg/day for benzyl alcohol (range 0.6–319.5 mg/kg/day) and 204.9 mg/kg/day (range 17.3–9,472.7) for propylene glycol [22].

Very recently (2012), a national survey on the extent of exposure was reported from Estonia [50]. During a 6-month interval and based on 1961 prescriptions for 107 different formulations (both enteral and parenteral formulations), the exposure of 348/490 neonates to 123 excipients was documented, of which 47 (38%) were classified as 'toxic or potentially toxic' to neonates. Almost all neonates (97%) were exposed to at least one of these 'toxic or potentially toxic' excipients after they had received both enteral or parenteral formulations [50]. Despite the fact that 19 formulations were licensed for use in neonates, about half of the formulations contained at least one potential harmful excipient. Parabens and sodium metabisulphite were the most commonly administered 'toxic or potential toxic' excipients that were administered in this Estonian cohort, while exposure to sodium benzoate, benzyl alcohol, propylene glycol, polysorbate 80 and ethanol was also documented [50].

Exposure to parabens and sodium metabisulphite in this specific cohort of neonates seemed to be related to a specific gentamicin formulation that was available in Estonia. The authors mentioned that the information that is currently mentioned on the summary of product characteristics (SPC) is not always complete (e.g. those on the concentrations of specific excipients in a given formulation). In fact, the amount of excipients in a specific formulation was only mentioned in 2/19 SPC documents that were approved for use in (pre)term neonates [50, 51], confirming the difficulties in retrieving the exact amounts of propylene glycol in intravenous formulations that are currently administered to newborn infants [23].

Although exposure to potential harmful excipients in the Estonian cohort (68%) [50, 51] was even more common when compared to that of a similar study from the Netherlands (52% for oral liquids, 7% for parenteral formulations) [52], both studies and the earlier-mentioned papers of Whitakker et al. and Shehab et al. suggest that excipient exposure is common, difficult to quantify and, in part, relates to the available country- or unit-specific formulations [12, 22, 50–52]. As mentioned by Lass et al., the gentamicin-associated paraben exposure in the Estonian cohort could have potentially been avoided because a paraben-free formulation is also available in Europe [50, 51]. Similarly, Van Riet-Nales et al. documented that for oral formulations containing potential harmful excipients, an alternative formulation with the same active compound but without such excipients was available in 22% of the formulations [52].

To further illustrate this diversity for both parenteral and enteral formulations, we provide some information on different phenobarbital formulations for parenteral ad-

Table 3. Different formulations containing phenobarbital as a sodium salt for intravenous administration

Vial	Excipient, concentration
30 mg/ml	ethanol 10%, propylene glycol 75%
60 mg/ml	ethanol 10%, propylene glycol 75%
65 mg/ml	ethanol 10%, benzyl alcohol 0.15%, propylene glycol 67.8%
130 mg/ml	ethanol 10%, propylene glycol 67.8%
200 mg/ml	ethanol 10%, propylene glycol 70%
250 mg/vial	Sodium phenobarbital, lyophilised, 'no additives'

When converted to an exposure ratio (mg propylene glycol/mg phenobarbital), there is a 5-fold difference between the different formulations.

ministration in neonates (table 3) that were retrieved from the literature. These findings further illustrate the available formulations and the formulation-specific exposure to different excipients that is likely influenced by local practices. Depending on the formulation used, there is a 5-fold difference in the propylene glycol exposure for every milligram of phenobarbital administered. Even more intriguing, there is a recent report on a propylene glycol-free formulation for intravenous phenobarbital administration that has been evaluated in terms of its safety and tolerance in neonates [53].

A Roadmap Towards Tailored Drug Administration in Neonates: A Subjective Opinion

We aim to provide a roadmap to further improve formulations and additives for neonates. In our opinion, improvements should focus on the need for tailored vials, and these studies should include a systematic search on excipient exposure in neonates. Meanwhile, prospective studies on the threshold of excipient tolerance in neonates should be stimulated. Finally, improved validation of extemporaneous formulation practices is needed because extemporaneous formulations will remain the final back up until age-appropriate formulations become available.

The Need for an Appropriate Balance between Dose, Volume and Drug Manipulations

Children should be treated with medicinal products of which the pharmaceutical design is tailored for use in the target-age group [54–57]. Neonates pose specific characteristics and needs; volume overload should be avoided, while too-low volumes might result in additional dose inaccuracy, irrespective of the type of formulation. This needs a balanced approach. Serial dilutions in order to achieve the required dose should be avoided because they are prone to errors, while such errors can be avoided by providing appropriate concentrations based on a dedicated, population-specific formulation [58, 59]. A recent illustration of such an approach is the development of a specific caffeine-containing vial for the treatment of apnoea of prematurity (20 mg/ml of caffeine citrate, equal to 10 mg/ml of caffeine base) that can be used for both parenteral as well as enteral administration.

Nunn et al. recently quantified the requirement for the manipulation of medicines to provide accurate doses for children, including neonates [60]. Over a 5-day period, 5,375 drug-administration events were recorded in neonatal and paediatric inpatients in one regional children's hospital. Despite this setting, about 10% of the patients was still judged to require manipulation or a small volume (<0.2 ml) of the medicine. Measured doses below 0.1 ml (either oral or intravenous) accounted for 25% of the manipulations, and the most common (60%) were in the neonatal intensive care unit [60]. The same research group described the development of a systematic review protocol to map the evidence related to drug manipulations conducted to obtain the required dose [61]. This was performed with the overall goal of improving the knowledge on the widespread practice of medicine manipulations because there was no easily accessible guidance for nurses or caregivers advising how medications could be safely manipulated to obtain the required dose. In essence, the authors illustrated that the most important hurdle was the absence of accepted terminology to describe all drug manipulations [11, 36, 60, 61].

Tailored vials for intravenous administration, resulting in appropriate, flexible and correct dosage of drugs in neonates, are needed. Besides the fact that 10-fold errors are more common when 'highly' concentrated formulations are used, there are also dilution-related errors that result in dosing inaccuracy [54, 57, 58, 62]. A recent illustration of the impact of the introduction of an inappropriate vial on dosing errors in neonates with subsequent relevant morbidity and mortality is the intravenous paracetamol formulation. Based on a 10-mg/ml paracetamol formulation in either a 50- or 100-ml vial, Dart and Rumack reported incidences of the 'famous' 10-fold errors and confirmed that these errors were most common in neonates and infants in the United States [63]. This finding confirmed those of other case reports or case series from the United Kingdom [63].

The impact of a 'paediatric vial' on dose accuracy has also been quantified in neonates [64]. Using population pharmacokinetics in a cohort of 254 preterm neonates, the unexplained variability in amikacin clearance in neonates, in part, was related to the vial used. A paediatric vial (50 mg/ml, 2 ml) resulted in an 8% reduction in unexplained variability when compared to an adult vial (250 mg/ml, 2 ml). Taking the amikacin dose (15–20 mg/kg) commonly administered in neonates into account, a 250-mg/ml formulation necessitates consecutive dilutions, which introduces additional dilution-related errors [64]. In essence, this observation illustrates the impact of consecutive dilutions on dose inaccuracy. Unfortunately, the need for consecutive dilutions of vials initially marketed for use in adults is a common practice [58, 60, 63,

Table 4. The reference doses (e.g. mg or mg/kg) in neonates were compared to the available, intravenous formulations to illustrate the need for sequential dilutions

Formulation	Concentration/volume	Units
Amikacin, adult vial	500 mg/2 ml	15–20 mg/kg
Amikacin, paediatric vial	100 mg/2 ml	15–20 mg/kg
Enoxaparin	40 mg/0.4 ml	1 mg/kg
Erythromycin	1,000 mg/20 ml	5–10 mg/kg
Fentanyl	100 µg/2 ml	1–3 µg/kg
Insulin	300 E/3 ml	0.1–1 E/kg/h
Midazolam	15 mg/3 ml	0.05–0.1 mg/kg
Paracetamol/acetaminophen	500 mg/50 ml	10 mg/kg
Phenobarbital	200 mg/1 ml	5 mg/kg
Propofol	200 mg/20 ml	1–3 mg/kg
Ranitidine	50 mg/2 ml	0.5–1 mg/kg

The formulations (alphabetical) are reported as they are available in Belgium, and this does not necessary reflect the setting in another country.

64]. This is further illustrated in table 4, where reference doses (e.g. mg or mg/kg) in neonates are compared to the available formulations.

Oral administration can be achieved by using several forms of dosage. However, because of the need for dosing flexibility and the inability to swallow solid-unit dosage forms, oral liquid formulations (e.g. syrup, liquid drops) are preferred in neonates and young infants [42]. Specific issues that need to be considered are the impact of tube feeding or simultaneous administration with milk on the bioavailability of the pharmaceutical product. For oral drugs commonly administered by a feeding tube (e.g. in preterm neonates), issues related to particle size, viscosity, dosing volume and compatibility with the tube material should be considered [42, 48].

The Need to Quantify and Limit Excipient Exposure

We need to learn more on the appropriateness of the established excipient use in neonatal drug formulations [36]. We hereby have to keep in mind that the currently authorised medicinal products with given excipients do not necessary reflect the gold standard, nor does this validate the unrestricted use of the same excipient in another formulation [14, 36, 37, 55].

We have already referred to two illustrative cases to raise the reader's awareness on this issue. Although exposure to gentamicin commonly results in co-exposure to parabens and/or sodium metabisulphite, a preservative-free formulation is available on the European market [50, 51]. Similarly, phenobarbital formulations for intravenous use commonly contain propylene glycol and/or ethanol (table 3), while the pharmacokinetic properties of a propylene glycol-free formulation and its effects on neonates has been tested [53]. The simultaneous availability of both thimerosal-containing and thimerosal-free formulations for vaccines in neonates is another reflection of the current variability and the need for further product improvements [29–33].

The acceptability of a given excipient in a medicinal product should be based on the overall risk-to-benefit evaluation of the product itself. In the case of the use of an excipient with an identified risk, the added value of the chosen pharmaceutical formulation should be considered [9, 40, 42]. This means that when compared with other pharmaceutical formulations for the same therapeutic compound but without these toxic excipients, the more appropriate formulation should be preferred. The same holds true for colorants or flavours. Similarly, new excipients without any evidence on their safety or tolerance in neonates should be introduced very cautiously and should necessitate a balanced decision based upon the potential risks versus benefits.

At best, this should be part of an integrated benefit/risk approach towards selecting the appropriate pharmaceutical dosage form. A structured framework for assessing the comparative benefits and risks of pharmaceutical design options with issues related to efficacy, safety and patient access to paediatric-dosage-form selection has recently been published [65].

The Need for Focused Studies on the Clinical Pharmacology of Excipients in Neonates
Recently initiated and on-going collaborative research initiatives to ameliorate access to information on excipients in neonates (STEP database, i.e. Safety and Toxicity of Excipients for Paediatrics database) [66] or to generate new information (ESNEE research initiative, European Study for Neonatal Excipient Exposure) on the epidemiology and tolerance of excipients are very useful approaches [67, 68].

Excipient safety data are available in peer-reviewed scientific journals, government reports and protected databases, but there is very limited access to paediatric data for the development of paediatric medicines [9, 17, 66]. Furthermore, these data are distributed over many sources, the available safety data have never been incorporated into a single comprehensive and readily accessible database, and some stakeholders consider some information as protected. Access to and organization of this data is the aim of the STEP database [66]. Neither regulatory agencies nor the pharmaceutical industry have a single central source of safety data on which to base decisions regarding safety and the need for additional studies. A database that provides manufacturers a basis for screening and selecting excipients for use in paediatric product development can, consequently, facilitate further product-specific safety, but toxicity studies are urgently needed [66].

The European Paediatric Formulation Initiative took the initiative, with the support of the FDA, European Medicines Agency and pharmaceutical industry, to collect retrievable information on excipients and to develop the STEP database. In addition to some more specific, manufacturer-related aims, the major aims of this initiative were (1) to conduct a high-level scientific literature review of the pharmacology, toxicology and safety data of a selected group of excipients that is used in or aimed for paediatric formulations, (2) to help determine the relationship between exposure and evidence of clinically significant toxicity in the paediatric age group or in specific paediatric subpopulations, and (3) to identify knowledge gaps and needed studies or provide the basis for the development of hypothesis-driven safety or toxicity studies [66].

The European Study for Neonatal Excipient Exposure (ESNEE) research initiative has been funded by ERA-NET PRIOMEDCHILD, a multinational, European research initiative with a specific focus on developmental clinical pharmacology [67, 68]. As described by the core research group, this initiative aims to develop a platform for the systematic assessment of excipients in neonates. The first step of this program is to establish which excipients are in use and how much of each excipient is included in medicines given to neonates, thus *'setting the scene'*. A pan-European survey is underway. The preliminary results with the key difficulties will be presented. The major challenge has been accessing data about excipients in existing medicines [67, 68]. The earlier-described data on the exposure to excipients from Estonia are the first observations related to this ESNEE research initiative [50, 51].

A second step of this ESNEE program is to determine what is known about the effects of excipients in neonates and juvenile animals. To do so, the research initiative is developing a series of systematic reviews about excipient toxicity. The preliminary results will be presented together with important issues on the design and analysis of a systematic review of this nature, i.e. *'knowledge collection and identifying missing links'* [67, 68].

The third step of the program is to measure the systemic concentrations of key excipients in neonates using dry blood spots and plasma samples in order to *'generate information on missing links'*. The final step of the ESNEE program is to integrate the work from the other steps into a systematic assessment of safety for each excipient, thus *'coming back to the clinical relevance'*. A generic framework for the assessment of excipient safety in neonates will be developed with the aim to illustrate how this can be applied by prescribers, pharmacists, manufacturers and regulatory agencies [67, 68].

Propylene glycol serves as a case study with reference to other excipients. We recently published our experiences on the feasibility and methodology applied to evaluate the pharmacokinetics and pharmacodynamics of propylene glycol [23]. This approach included population pharmacokinetics modelling, systematic collection of clinical observations and comparison of excipient-exposed compared to non-excipient-exposed neonates [23–25].

Validation of Compounding Practices for Drug Formulations in Neonates

It may not always be possible to provide authorised, commercially manufactured, ready-to-administer preparations for use in neonates. Commonly, economic constraints mean that marketed formulations do not meet the specific requirements of all patient groups, which is commonly applicable for neonates (formulation and dose). As a consequence, it is anticipated that compounding practices will remain common [69–73]. Since the process of compounding is not without risks, the first intent of the manufacturer should be to provide an age-appropriate formulation. An alternative could be that the manufacturer provides evidence on the appropriate reconstitution or compounding of a given formulation. Such available evidence can subsequently be converted to instructions for reconstitution, compounding or manipulation and can be provided in the SPC. A recent illustration of such an approach is the compounding of an oral solution of valganciclovir for use in neonates and infants with CMV infection [74].

Unfortunately, non-authorised (i.e. information not included in the SPC) compounding or manipulation is still very common, although the quality of compounding and of excipient ingredients may vary considerably. This non-authorised approach may facilitate the use of a given drug in neonates but is unlicensed and obviously carries risks of patient safety related to the quality of the formulation, the bioavailability of the compound and the excipients used for compounding [69–73].

In an effort to improve the practice on extemporaneous dispensing, the WHO commissioned a literature review and development of guidelines on extemporaneous dispensing. Despite some relevant concerns on the risks of inappropriate preparations and the risk of diverting efforts to improve formulation availability in an attempt to re-introduce the practice of compounding available adult dosage forms for use in children, a document describing this practice has been published on the WHO website. It should hereby be re-emphasized that compounding remains the 'last resort' [75].

The need for validation of such compounding practices has been nicely illustrated in the design and evaluation of a paediatric oral formulation with a low concentration of hydrochlorothiazide that is suitable for use in neonates. Santovena et al. documented that of 5 evaluated suspensions of hydrochlorothiazide (2 mg/ml), only one guaranteed the correct dose administration and stability after 3-week, light-protected storage at 5°C [76].

Conclusion: Neonates Are in Need of Tailored Drug Development

Excipients in Neonatal Drug Formulations: Friend and Foe?

Children display maturation in drug disposition, but this is most prominent in early infancy. Although the principles of drug disposition also apply to neonates, their specific characteristics warrant a focused assessment. As a consequence, neonates are in need of tailored drug development, and clinical research should hereby focus on both new as well as already-existing compounds. Good prescribing involves assurance that the administered drug is of sufficient pharmaceutical quality, that an appropriate formulation is used, and that there is sufficient knowledge on the pharmacokinetics, pharmacodynamics and safety of the administered compound. For an extensive review on the issues of developmental pharmacokinetics and the integration of pharmacokinetics and pharmacodynamics, we refer to Chapters 3 and 4 of this issue, while this chapter on neonatal formulations and additives mainly focuses on issues related to the appropriateness of a given formulation.

We hereby aimed to stress that tailored, personalized clinical pharmacology for neonates related to neonatal formulations and additives with different case reports on toxicity [77–80] in addition to the earlier reported case series [18–36] need to be considered. Further progress can be made through collaborative efforts between industry, caregivers, academia and regulatory agencies that should focus on product availability (tailored formulations), knowledge integration of currently available information, making such information accessible, validating the assumed safety of the currently used excipients, and validating procedures and practices on compounding [36, 42, 48, 55, 81].

Acknowledgements

Karel Allegaert is supported by the Fund for Scientific Research, Flanders (Fundamental Clinical Investigatorship 1800209N). The clinical research of J.N. van den Anker is supported by NIH (5R01HD048689; 5K24DA027992; 5R01HD060543; 5U54). The authors have no conflict of interest to report.

References

1 Kearns GL, Abdel-Rahman SM, Alander SW, et al: Developmental pharmacology: drug disposition, action, and therapy in infants and children. N Engl J Med 2003;349:1157–1167.

2 Jacqz-Aigrain E: Drug policy in Europe research and funding in neonates: current challenges, future perspectives, new opportunities. Early Hum Dev 2011; 87(suppl 1):S27–S30.

3 Allegaert K, Verbesselt R, Naulaers G, et al: Developmental pharmacology: neonates are not just small adults. Acta Clin Belg 2008;63:16–24.

4 Fanos V, Yurdakok M: Personalized neonatal medicine. J Matern Fetal Neonatal Med 2010;23(suppl 3):4–6.

5 Van den Anker J: Managing drugs safely. Semin Fetal Neonatal Med 2005;10:73–81.

6 Allegaert K, Langhendries JP, van den Anker JN: Educational paper: do we need neonatal clinical pharmacologists? Eur J Pediatr 2013;172:429–435.

7 Van den Anker J, Allegaert K: Clinical pharmacology in neonates and young infants: the benefit of a population-tailored approach. Expert Rev Clin Pharmacol 2012;5:5–8.

8 Nahata MC: Safety of 'inert' additives or excipients in paediatric medicines. Arch Dis Child Fetal Neonatal Ed 2009;94:F392–F393.

9 Fabiano V, Mameli C, Zuccotti GV: Paediatric pharmacology: remember the excipients. Pharmacol Res 2011;63:362–365.

10 Knoppert DC: Pediatric formulations: international issues and potential solutions. Paediatr Drugs 2009; 11:55–56.

11 Ernest TB, Elder DP, Martini LG, et al: Developing paediatric medicines: identifying the needs and recognizing the challenges. J Pharm Pharmacol 2007; 59:1043–1055.

12 Whittaker A, Currie AE, Turner MA, et al: Toxic additives in medication for preterm infants. Arch Dis Child Fetal Neonatal Ed 2009;94:F236-F240.

13 Nahata MC, Allen LV Jr: Extemporaneous drug formulations. Clin Ther 2008;30:2112–2119.

14 Turner MA, Lewis S, Hawcutt DB, et al: Prioritising neonatal medicines research: UK Medicines for Children Research Network scoping survey. BMC Pediatr 2009;9:50.

15 Sam T, Ernest TB, Walsh J, et al. A benefit/risk approach towards selecting appropriate pharmaceutical dosage forms – an application for paediatric dosage form selection. Int J Pharm 2012;435:115–123.

16 Wille D, Hauri-Hohl M, Vonbach P, et al: Too much of too little: xylitol, an unusual trigger of a chronic metabolic hyperchloremic acidosis. Eur J Pediatr 2010;169:1549–1551.

17 American Academy of Pediatrics, Committee on Drugs: Inactive ingredients in pharmaceutical products: update (subject review). Pediatrics 1997;99: 268–278.

18 Gershanik J, Boecler B, Ensley H, et al: The gasping syndrome and benzyl alcohol poisoning. N Engl J Med 1982;307:1384–1388.

19 LeBel M, Ferron L, Masson M, et al: Benzyl alcohol metabolism and elimination in neonates. Dev Pharmacol Ther 1988;11:347–456.

20 Jardine DS, Rogers K: Relationship of benzyl alcohol to kernicterus, intraventricular haemorrhage, and mortality in preterm infants. Pediatrics 1989;83: 153–160.
21 Brown WJ, Buist NR, Gipson HT, et al: Fatal benzyl alcohol poisoning in a neonatal intensive care unit. Lancet 1982;8283:1250.
22 Shehab N, Lewis CL, Streetman DD, et al: Exposure to the pharmaceutical excipients benzyl alcohol and propylene glycol among critically ill neonates. Pediatr Crit Care Med 2009;10:256–259.
23 Kulo A, de Hoon J, Allegaert K: The propylene glycol research project to illustrate the feasibility and difficulties to study toxicokinetics in neonates. Int J Pharm 2012;435:112–114.
24 Allegaert K, Vanhaesebrouck S, Kulo A, et al: Prospective assessment of short-term propylene glycol tolerance in neonates. Arch Dis Child 2010;95:1054–1058.
25 De Cock RF, Knibbe CA, Kulo A, et al: Developmental pharmacokinetics of propylene glycol in preterm and term neonates. Br J Clin Pharmacol 2013;75: 162–171.
26 MacDonald MG, Fletcher AB, Johnson EL, et al: The potential toxicity to neonates of multivitamin preparations used in parenteral nutrition. JPEN J Parenter Enteral Nutr 1987;11:169–171.
27 MacDonald MH, Getson PR, Glasgow AM, et al: Propylene glycol: increased incidence of seizures in low birth weight infants. Pediatrics 1987;79:622–625.
28 Lopinavir + ritonavir oral solution: dangerous form for newborns. Prescrire Int 2011;20:237.
29 Ball LK, Ball R, Pratt RD: An assessment of thimerosal use in childhood vaccines. Pediatrics 2001;107: 1147–1154.
30 Dorea JG, Bezerra VL, Fajon V, et al: Speciation of methyl- and ethyl-mercury in hair of breastfed infants acutely exposed to thimerosal-containing vaccines. Clin Chim Acta 2011;412:1563–1566.
31 Price CS, Thompson WW, Goodson B, et al: Prenatal and infant exposure to thimerosal from vaccines and immunoglobulins and risk of autism. Pediatrics 2010;126:656–664.
32 Thompson WW, Price C, Goodson B, et al: Early thimerosal exposure and neuropsychological outcomes at 7 to 10 years. N Engl J Med 2007;357:1281–1292.
33 Badger J, Kubusek J, Hayney MS: Safety of adjuvants and excipients in vaccines. J Am Pharm Assoc 2009; 49:826–827.
34 Mrozek-Budzyn D, Majewska R, Kieltyka A, et al: Neonatal exposure to Thimerosal from vaccines and child development in the first 3 years of life. Neurotoxicol Teratol 2012;34:592–597.
35 Zuccotti GV, Fabiano V: Safety issues with ethanol as an excipient in drugs intended for pediatric use. Expert Opin Drug Saf 2011;10:499–502.
36 Turner MA: Neonatal drug development. Early Hum Dev 2011;87:763–768.
37 Tuleu C, Breitkreutz J: Formulation related issues in paediatric clinical pharmacology. Eur J Pediatr 2013; 172:717–720.
38 Ursino MG, Poluzzi E, Caramella C, et al: Excipients in medicinal products used in gastroenterology as a possible cause of side effects. Regul Toxicol Pharmacol 2011;60:93–105.
39 What are excipients doing in medical products? Drug Ther Bull 2009;47:81–84.
40 Walsch J: Excipients for the formulation of medicines for children. Eur Indust Pharm 2012;13:14–16.
41 Hamman J, Steenekamp J: Excipients with specialized functions for effective drug delivery. Expert Opin Drug Deliv 2012;9:219–230.
42 http://www.ema.europa/docs/en_GB/document_library/Scientific_guideline/2009/09/WC500003750.pdf. Guideline on the investigation of medicinal products in the term and preterm neonate (latest access October 2012).
43 Adkin DA, Davis SS, Sparrow RA, et al: The effects of pharmaceutical excipients on small intestinal transit. Br J Clin Pharmacol 1995;39:381–387.
44 Turkova A, Roilides E, Sharland M: Amphotericin B in neonates: deoxycholate or lipid formulation as first-line therapy – is there a 'right' choice? Curr Opin Infect Dis 2011;24:163–171.
45 Kasirye P, Kendall L, Adkison KK, et al: Pharmacokinetics of antiretroviral drug varies with formulation in the target population of children with HIV-1. Clin Pharmacol Ther 2012;91:272–280.
46 Chen H, Spagnoli F, Burris M, et al: Nanoerythropoietin is 10-times more effective than regular erythropoietin in neuroprotection in a neonatal rat model of hypoxia and ischemia. Stroke 2012;43:884–887.
47 Vesikari T, Knuf M, Wutzler P, et al: Oil-in-water emulsion adjuvant with influenza vaccine in young children. N Engl J Med 2011;365:1406–1416.
48 http://www.ema.europa.eu/docs/en_GB/document_library/Scientific_guideline/2011/06/WC500107908.pdf. Guideline on pharmaceutical development of medicines for paediatric use (draft) (latest access October 2012).
49 Giacoia GP, Birenbaum DL, Sachs HC, et al: The newborn drug development initiative. Pediatrics 2006;117:S1–S8.
50 Lass J, Käär R, Jõgi K, et al: Drug utilisation pattern and off-label use of medicines in Estonian neonatal units. Eur J Clin Pharmacol 2011;67:1263–1271.
51 Lass J, Naelapaa K, Shah U, et al: Hospitalised neonates in Estonia commonly receive potentially harmful excipients. BMC Pediatr 2012;12:136.
52 Van Riet-Nales DA, de Jager KE, Schobben AF, et al: The availability and age-appropriateness of medicines authorized for children in The Netherlands. Br J Clin Pharmacol 2011;72:465–473.

53 Kawada K, Itoh S, Itani Y, et al: A clinical trial assessing the efficacy and safety of a new injectable formula of sodium phenobarbital containing no additives for the treatment of neonatal seizures. Jpn J Clin Pharmacol Ther 2011;42:205–210.
54 Uppal N, Yasseen B, Seto W, et al: Drug formulations that require less than 0.1 mL of stock solution to prepare doses for infants and children. CMAJ 2011; 183:E246–E248.
55 Rieder M: If children ruled the pharmaceutical industry: the need for pediatric formulations. Drug News Perspect 2010;23:458–464.
56 Caldwell NA, Rackham O: Children's doses should be measurable. Arch Dis Child 2010;95:313.
57 Broussard L: Small size, big risk: preventing neonatal and pediatric medication errors. Nurs Womens Health 2010;14:405–408.
58 Rosenbluth G, Wilson SD: Pediatric and neonatal patients are particularly vulnerable to epinephrine dosing errors. Ann Emerg Med 2010;56:704–705; author reply 705.
59 Dessi A, Salemi C, Fanos V, et al: Drug treatments in a neonatal setting: focus on the off-label use in the first month of life. Pharm World Sci 2010;32:120–124.
60 Nunn A, Craig JV, Shah UU, et al: Estimating the requirement for manipulation of medicines to provide accurate doses for children. Eur J Hosp Pharm 2013;20:3–7.
61 Richey RH, Craig JV, Shah UU, et al: The manipulation of drugs to obtain the required dose: systematic review. J Adv Nurs 2012;68:2103–2112.
62 Donnell C, Nunn T: How to manipulate drugs so they can be given to children. Nurs Child Young People 2011;23:6–7.
63 Dart RC, Rumack BH: Intravenous acetaminophen in the United States: iatrogenic dosing errors. Pediatrics 2012;129:349–353.
64 Allegaert K, Anderson BJ, Vrancken M, et al: Impact of a paediatric vial on the magnitude of systematic medication errors in neonates. Paediatr Perinat Drug Ther 2006;7:59–63.
65 Ernest TB, Craig J, Nunn A, et al: Preparation of medicines for children – a hierarchy of classification. Int J Pharm 2012;435:124–130.
66 Salunke S, Giacoia G, Tuleu C: The STEP (Safety and Toxicity of Excipients for Paediatrics) database. Par 1 – A need assessment study. Int J Pharm 2012;435: 101–111.
67 Turner MA, Storme T: European study of neonatal excipient exposure (ESNEE). Eur J Hosp Pharm 2012;19:67.
68 http://www.esnee.eu. (latest access October 2012).
69 Conroy S: Extemporaneous (magistral) preparation of oral medicines for children in European hospitals. Acta Paediatr 2003;92:408–410.
70 Brion F, Nunn AJ, Rieutord A: Extemporaneous (magistral) preparation of oral medicines for children in European hospitals. Acta Paediatr 2003;92: 486–490.
71 Kairuz T, Chhim S, Hasan F, et al: Extemporaneous compounding in a sample of New Zealand hospitals: a retrospective survey. Z Med J 2007;120:U2466.
72 Dickinson CJ, Wagner DS, Shaw BE, et al: A systematic approach to improving medication safety in a pediatric intensive care unit. Crit Care Nurs Q 2012; 35:15–26.
73 Yin HS, Wolf MS, Dreyer BP, et al: Evaluation of consistency in dosing directions and measuring devices for pediatric non-prescription liquid medications. JAMA 2010;304:2595–2602.
74 Acosta EP, Brundage RC, King JR: Ganciclovir population pharmacokinetics in neonates following intravenous administration of ganciclovir and oral administration of a liquid valganciclovir formulation. Clin Pharmacol Ther 2007;81:867–872.
75 Breitkreutz J: European perspectives on pediatric formulations. Clin Ther 2008;30:2146–2154.
76 Santovena A, Hernandeze-Paiz Z, Farina JB: Design of a pediatric oral formulation with a low proportion of hydrochlorothiazide. Int J Pharm 2012;423:360–364.
77 Genuini M, Freihuber C, Girard I, et al: Neonatal intoxication with pyrimethamine: risk due to the absence of pediatric formulation? Arch Pediatr 2011; 18:1084–1086.
78 Masi S, de Cléty SC, Anslot C, et al: Acute amiodarone toxicity due to an administration error: could excipient be responsible? Br J Clin Pharmacol 2009; 67:691–693.
79 Hall CM, Milligan DW, Berrington J: Probable adverse reaction to a pharmaceutical excipient. Arch Dis Child Fetal Neonatal Ed 2004;89:F184.
80 Lesko SM, Mitchell AA: Total bilirubin level in relation to excipients in parenteral morphine sulfate administered to seriously ill newborn infants. Paediatr Perinat Epidemiol 1994;8:401–410.
81 http://www.eupfi.org/gpage11.html. (latest access October 2012).

Karel Allegaert, MD, PhD
Neonatal Intensive Care Unit, University Hospital
Herestraat 49
BE–3000 Leuven (Belgium)
E-Mail karel.allegaert@uzleuven.be

Mimouni FB, van den Anker JN (eds): Neonatal Pharmacology and Nutrition Update.
Pediatr Adolesc Med. Basel, Karger, 2015, vol 18, pp 58–69 (DOI: 10.1159/000365025)

Modelling and Simulation to Support Neonatal Clinical Trials

Feras Khalil · Stephanie Läer

Department of Clinical Pharmacy and Pharmacotherapy, Heinrich-Heine University of Düsseldorf, Düsseldorf, Germany

Abstract

Modelling and simulation are acknowledged methodologies used by industry, academia, and regulatory agencies to support and optimize clinical trials and are used as data-analysis tools during various stages of the drug-development process. Conventional modelling and simulation tools are data driven, and besides their potential in clinical applications, particularly in establishing therapeutic dosage regimens and addressing factors responsible for the observed variability in drug behaviour in a certain population, these tools are unsuitable for use beyond the experimental data, e.g., for age extrapolation to neonates. In contrast, physiology-based pharmacokinetic (PBPK) models are mechanistic models that are independent of the measured concentrations and are based instead on the known anatomy and physiology of the living organism being modelled. They can also be used as a predictive tool to explore the changes in drug behaviour a priori, e.g., for age extrapolation, and are considered to be superior to classical compartmental models in this respect. This report will explore the potential contributions of PBPK models to paediatric and neonatal clinical trials, will give a brief overview of the basic concepts of PBPK modelling and, where it is appropriate, will provide an overview of examples of such models reported in the published literature.

Introduction

Modelling and simulation are acknowledged methodologies used by industry, academia, and regulatory agencies to support and optimize clinical trials and are used as data-analysis tools during various stages of the drug-development process [1–3]. Although the terms modelling and simulation are closely related, modelling is the science of using mathematical language to describe and quantify a system or a process, whereas simulation refers to the use of these models to make quantitative predictions [4]. In the field of pharmacokinetics (PKs), one has to differentiate between conventional PK compartmental modelling and physiologically based pharmacokinetic modelling (PBPK). Both methodologies can be extended to incorporate a pharmacodynamic component and thus link drug exposure with a certain effect.

Conventional PK compartmental models have important clinical applications, particularly in establishing therapeutic dosage regimens and addressing factors responsible for the observed variability in drug behaviour in a certain population. However, since they are data driven (i.e., dependent with regard to their structure and parameters on the experimental data available), such models are inherently limited in the information they can provide. Moreover, they are not obviously related to the anatomical structure or the physiological function of the species under study. This makes these models unsuitable for use beyond the experimental data (e.g., for age extrapolation) or for exploring changes in drug PK under different physiological, pathological, or pharmacological conditions.

In contrast, PBPK models are mechanistic models that are independent of the measured concentrations and are based instead on the known anatomy and physiology of the living organism being modelled [5]. These models utilize actual measurements of the complex anatomical and physiological processes that are involved in absorption, distribution, metabolism, and excretion [5]. Such physiologically realistic models provide a rational basis for inter-species, inter-individual, or across-age scaling, and they are able to provide greater insights into drug disposition in the body because they can accurately describe fluctuations in drug concentrations in multiple body tissues over time. These models can also be used as predictive tools a priori to explore the changes in drug behaviour under altered physiological conditions or in pathological states. For these reasons, PBPK models are considered to be superior to classical compartmental models.

A combination of factors, including improvements in modelling software, a substantial increase in the availability of age-specific physiological data required for optimization of PBPK models, and increased awareness of and interest in paediatric research – especially after the new regulations on medicinal products for paediatric use in both the United States and the European Union went into effect – have together encouraged the utilization of PBPK models as tools to bridge paediatric and adult pharmacology over the past few years [6, 7]. In children, and specifically in neonates, many constraints exist and hinder the accurate measurement of in vivo drug concentrations, making any method capable of generating reliable information on drug exposure in this special population especially valuable.

In this chapter, we explore the potential contributions of PBPK models to paediatric and neonatal clinical trials. In this context, a quick overview of the basic concepts of PBPK modelling is appropriate and will be followed by an overview of examples of such models reported in the published literature.

Discussion

General Concepts and Methodology of Physiologically Based Pharmacokinetic Modelling

In PBPK modelling, physiological processes in the living organism being studied are simulated by representing various organs and tissues as compartments that are structurally connected via the blood circulation and mathematically connected by different mass-balance equations that utilize both physiological and compound-specific parameters [8]. The goal of such modelling practices is to quantitatively describe the fate of a drug in the body; therefore, a typical output is a set of predicted drug concentrations after a certain drug application, which could be obtained not only in the blood/plasma, but also in other tissues or organs. Figure 1 depicts a simplified scheme of the concept of PBPK modelling. A 'global' or 'whole-body' PBPK model includes almost all body organs and tissues in one way or another. However, it should be noted that not every PBPK model needs to include all body tissues. Available data on the anatomy and physiology of the biological system, the properties of the modelled drug, as well as the model's purpose will determine which tissues are appropriate for inclusion in the model structure.

As mentioned, equations that define the movement of the drug between the model compartments take into consideration both physiological and compound-dependent parameters. The physiological parameters account for the anatomical structure and physiological processes (e.g., cardiac output, organ/tissue volumes and blood flows, tissue composition, surface area, pH values, and/or transit times for the gastrointestinal tract) of the species being modelled. On the other hand, the compound-dependent parameters include, in addition to the physiochemical properties of the drug (e.g., molecular weight, lipophilicity, ionization, solubility, and plasma-protein binding), information such as the permeability and partitioning of the substance between body tissues and the blood/plasma. Also, included in modelling equations is a measure of drug clearance, which is both a compound- and species-specific parameter.

The PBPK model can be developed after deciding the general structure and collecting the necessary parameters. Several dedicated commercial software packages for developing PBPK models are available for this purpose. These packages fall into one of two principal categories: general mathematical and engineering modelling packages and specialized PBPK modelling software packages. Briefly, general modelling software packages (e.g., MATLAB®) provide a programming language for the model code, numerical solutions for the ordinary differential equations that define the system being modelled, and a graphical output of the simulation results. These software packages offer much flexibility to the model developer but require more advanced modelling and programming skills and experience. On the other hand, dedicated PBPK modelling software packages such as PK-Sim® [9] and Simcyp® [10] provide the researcher with an available model structure and a broad dataset of already incorporated physiological parameters but offer less flexibility in model development.

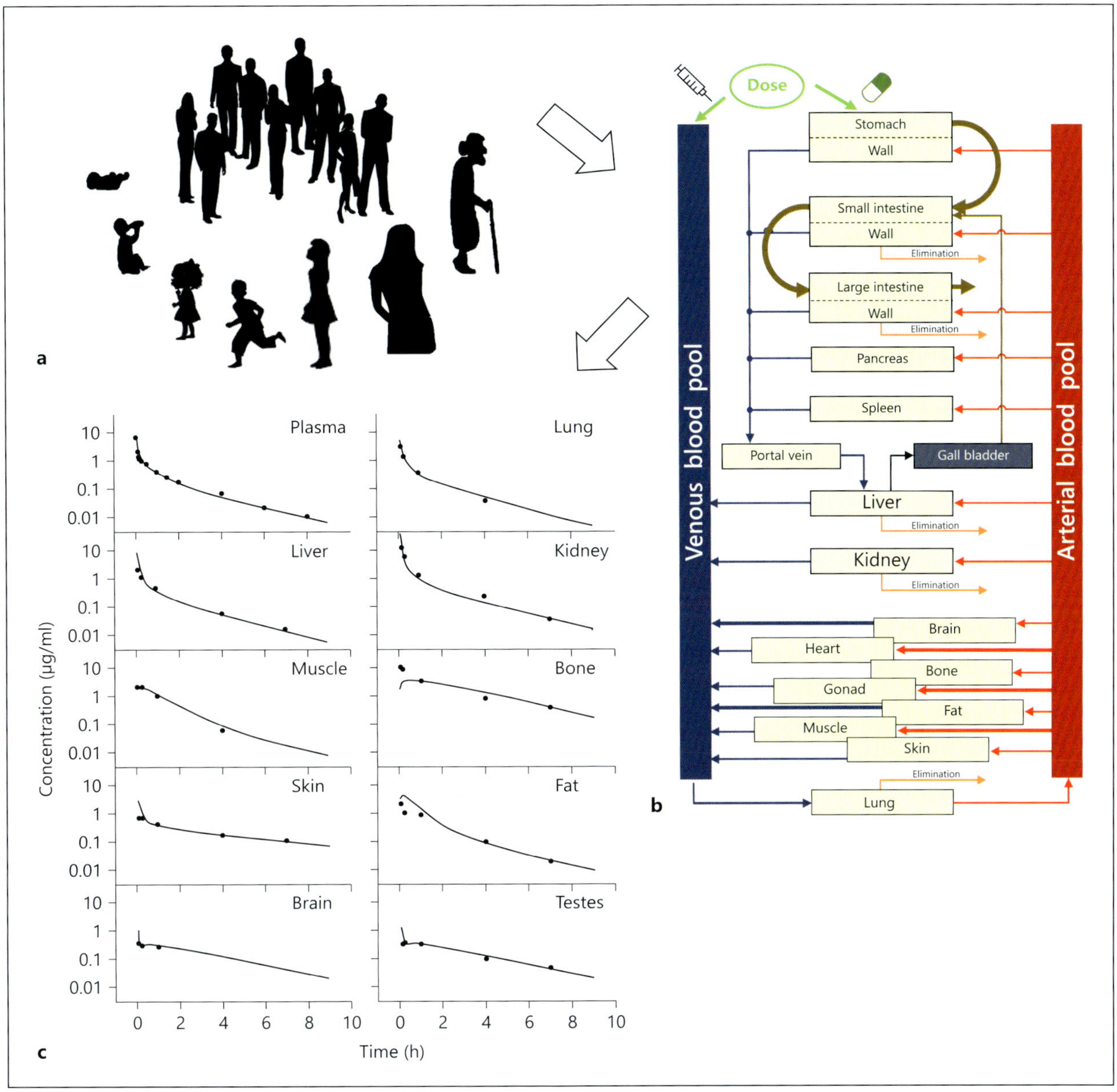

Fig. 1. The concept for building a PBPK model, adapted according to Willmann et al. [9]. **a** Organisms (e.g., humans of different ages or populations) are the basis for the model. **b** The organism is divided into a number of compartments, each representing a single organ. To describe the distribution of compounds in the body, the organs are connected via their arteries and veins to the arterial and venous blood pools. Inter-compartmental mass transport occurs via organ-specific blood flow rates, and the organs are mathematically connected. **c** Output of the model: concentration-time curves for the substances that are shown include simulated (lines) and observed (dots) ciprofloxacin concentrations in various organs after ciprofloxacin (5 mg/kg) was intravenously applied to a rat.

Many of these software packages also permit the simulation of virtual patient populations, such as obese or morbidly obese individuals and patients with renal impairment or liver cirrhosis, and include a clearance prediction model that incorporates knowledge of the growth, development, and maturation of various organs and tissues involved in drug metabolism and elimination across paediatric age groups to predict clearance in children on the basis of adult values [9, 10].

Potential Applications of Physiologically Based Pharmacokinetic Models in Paediatric Drug Development

There are many potential applications of PBPK models in paediatric trials and research [1, 4, 5]. The following section provides examples of the potential applications of PBPK models in paediatric drug research and discusses them in detail.

Using the Paediatric Physiologically Based Pharmacokinetic Model to Suggest Dosing in Children

An example of how a paediatric PBPK model can be used to suggest age-specific dosing for sildenafil has been presented by Hsien, who developed a PBPK model for sildenafil in adults using a specialized modelling software tool [11]. After validation of the basic PBPK model using adult data, it was extended to children using both data on age-specific physiological parameters that were embedded in the software and a clearance-scaling module – a module that takes into consideration the specific clearance pathways involved and their ontogeny – to predict the age-specific clearance of sildenafil. The paediatric model was used to predict plasma concentrations of sildenafil in virtual children. This data could supplement the scarce paediatric PK data available in the published literature. In a subsequent step, the paediatric PBPK model of sildenafil was used to run simulations in virtual paediatric populations of different ages to estimate drug exposure after administration of a weight-normalized dose comparable to that given to adults. The results of the simulations showed that after 3 months of age, exposure to the same weight-normalized dose increased with age of the children across the different paediatric age groups, suggesting that age-specific dose adaptation is necessary to achieve a relatively constant drug exposure in adults and children (fig. 2). The suggested dosing adjustments for the different paediatric age groups in this example of sildenafil are yet to be validated with prospectively collected data and are, therefore, currently hypothetical. Nevertheless, upon establishing and validating the use of PBPK modelling for this purpose, the provided data may help clinical trials become more 'confirmatory' rather than 'exploratory'. The modelling exercise will thus potentially save time and effort and decrease the number of trials needed to be performed using children.

Using the Paediatric Physiologically Based Pharmacokinetic Model to Suggest Sampling Times

Examples describing the use of a PBPK model to determine the optimal sampling times for paediatric studies have been reported [12, 13]. Willmann et al. compared

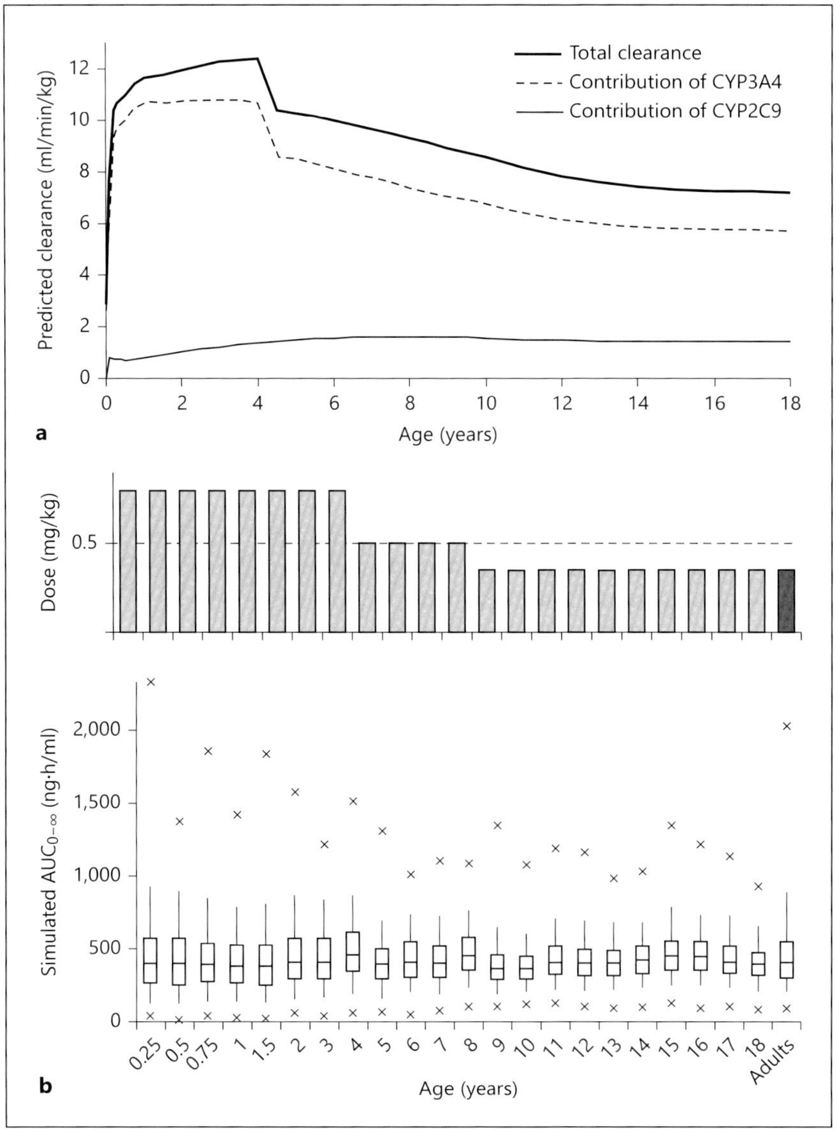

Fig. 2. Simulation results using the PK-Sim® software of a PBPK model for sildenafil in children [11]. **a** Predicted age-dependent sildenafil hepatic clearance across different paediatric ages based on the clearance-scaling module in the PK-Sim® software. **b** Age-related doses for oral sildenafil in children depending on the simulated age-related exposure (not shown) of sildenafil in a virtual paediatric population and the estimated exposure of the estimated doses of sildenafil in children between 3 months and 18 years. Potential paediatric doses based on simulations for sildenafil to achieve adult exposure: infants and children from 3 months to 4 years: 0.8 mg/kg; children from 5 to 8 years: 0.5 mg/kg; and children older than 8 years: 0.35 mg/kg, as in adults. The box plots represent the median, 25th and 75th percentiles (box), 5th and 95th percentiles (error bar), and maximum and minimum values (x) of $AUC_{0-\infty}$ from 1,000 simulations in each age group.

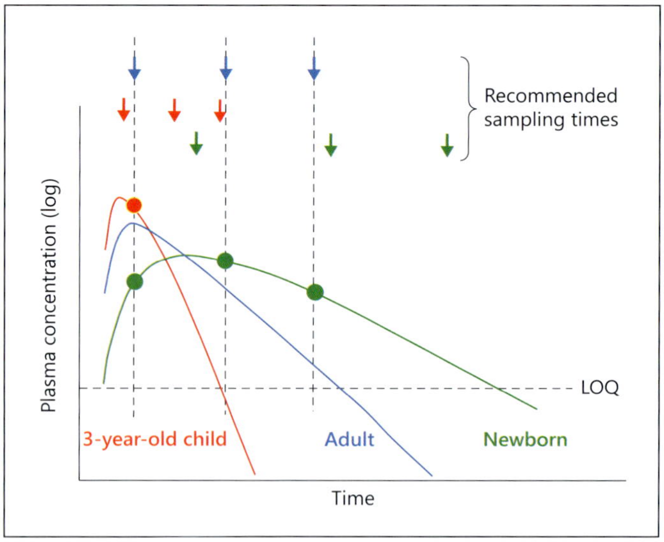

Fig. 3. Schematic drawing of a potential application of the PBPK simulation for children of different ages to find optimal blood-sampling time points for the PK investigations in a future paediatric trial according to Willmann [12]. Arrows indicate the optimal sampling time for a newborn, a 3-year-old, and an adult. LOQ = Limit of quantification.

the possible differences between suggested paediatric sampling times based on adult concentration-time data and suggested sampling times based on paediatric simulations performed using a PBPK model (fig. 3) [12]. As shown by the study, sampling times based on paediatric simulations performed using a PBPK model can potentially help detect the best sampling times for a PK analysis and thereby avoid having to take blood samples when the drug concentration is out of the range of detection. This is especially of great importance in neonates and infants because taking blood samples is more difficult than in adults and presents a significant challenge when conducting paediatric clinical trials. The primary reason for using a PBPK model to provide such information in advance is to help optimize the conduct of these trials. Whether these techniques can reduce the number of children required to be enrolled in clinical trials – thereby saving time, effort, and costs – remains to be determined.

Building a Paediatric Physiologically Based Pharmacokinetic Model to Predict Altered Drug Pharmacokinetics Due to Drug Interactions

Another publication has discussed multiple applications of PBPK models to predict drug PK in children under different conditions and to assess plasma:brain drug concentrations in children [14]. The authors performed multiple simulations that replicated actual paediatric clinical trials. One interesting example showed how a paediatric model could be used to simulate complex drug-drug interactions using the example of a 2-year-old child who was a patient in a paediatric intensive care unit (ICU) and received midazolam, among other drugs. The simulations were able to show the effect of the sequential addition of rifampicin (a CYP3A4 inducer), rifampicin and fluconazole (a CYP3A4 inhibitor), and rifampicin, fluconazole, and clarithromycin (a

Table 1. Reported physiology-based paediatric models in the literature that were evaluated using experimental data in children

Study	Modelled drugs	Type of drug application	Neonatal data included	Reference No.
Ginsberg et al., 2004	Caffeine and theophylline	intravenous	yes	[18]
Björkman, 2005	Theophylline and midazolam	intravenous	yes	[19]
Edginton et al., 2006	Paracetamol, alfentanil, morphine, theophylline, and levofloxacin	intravenous	yes	[20]
Johnson et al., 2010	Multiple, including: midazolam, ibuprofen, zolpidem, itraconazole, theophylline, and caffeine	intravenous and oral	no	[14]
Parrott et al., 2011	Oseltamivir and its active metabolite	oral	yes	[23]
Kersting et al., 2012	Etoposide	intravenous	no	[21]
Mahraj et al., 2012	Lorazepam	intravenous	no	[22]

CYP3A4 inhibitor) on the plasma concentrations of midazolam (a CYP3A4 substrate). This example illustrates the ability of PBPK modelling to evaluate complex drug-drug interactions and to explore 'what if' scenarios. As a next step, these models need to be validated by prospective PK data in children as an ultimate proof of their accuracy. Having thus qualified the models, 'what if' scenarios could be simulated to support future trial designs or even guide individual drug treatments.

As can be seen, there is enormous potential for the application of PBPK models in paediatric research and drug development. However, in order for these models to be practically implemented in neonatal clinical trials to predict drug exposure, to recommend dosing regimens, or to suggest optimal sampling times, a certain degree of confidence in the accuracy of their predictions must first be established. This confidence can be achieved by developing and reporting paediatric PBPK models that are validated using already available experimental data in order to judge whether their predictions are acceptable. The next section provides a quick overview of the current state of the literature pertaining to validated paediatric PBPK models.

Overview of Validated Paediatric Physiologically Based Pharmacokinetic Models Reported in the Published Literature

A few whole-body paediatric PBPK models that were validated using observed paediatric clinical data on intravenous or oral drug applications in humans have been published over the past few years. Table 1 summarizes the current state of the published literature on validated paediatric PBPK models. Models that were not validated with experimental paediatric data [13, 15] as well as publications that focused only on one aspect of the drug PKs (e.g., to predict only the clearance of the drugs) [16, 17] were not considered. Moreover, of the 6 reported paediatric whole-body

PBPK models [14, 18–22] that were validated with data on the intravenous application of 10 different drugs, only 3 models [18–20] included neonatal data in their evaluations. On the other hand, of the 2 publications [14, 23] reporting paediatric models evaluating the oral application of 6 drugs, only 1 included neonatal experimental data [23]. The absence of unified measures of model predictability and non-inclusion of neonatal data in a few instances made it difficult to compare the results of the different models. Nevertheless, a short summary of these models will be given below.

Ginsberg et al. published a paediatric model evaluating the disposition of caffeine and theophylline in neonates and adults after intravenous application in 2004 [18]. The model included age-specific data for the necessary physiological parameters (e.g., cardiac output, tissue/compartment volumes, blood flows, and clearance pathways) and compared predicted and observed clearance and half-life ($t_{1/2}$) values. The model predicted the clearance of caffeine in neonates less accurately than in adults (more than a 3-fold error in neonates vs less than a 2-fold error in adults), while the accuracy of the model for theophylline was almost identical for neonates and adults (a 2- to 3-fold error in both).

A second model was published by Björkman et al. shortly after the previous one [19]. Like the model published by Ginsberg et al., this model also incorporated age-specific values for the necessary physiological parameters. It was validated with adult and paediatric experimental data on intravenously administered theophylline and midazolam. All of the children were grouped together during model validation; therefore, a separate evaluation of the model predictions in neonates was not possible. However, this model was considered to appropriately predict clearance, volume of distribution (V_d), and $t_{1/2}$ for the whole simulated paediatric population.

Another model was reported by Edginton et al. 2 years later [20]. The authors extended an existing adult PBPK model by using age-related physiological parameters for children from birth to age 18 and combined this data with the age-specific predicted clearance. The model was then evaluated using adult and paediatric clinical data on the intravenous application of paracetamol, theophylline, levofloxacin, alfentanil, and morphine. The predicted plasma concentration-time curves, clearance, V_d, and $t_{1/2}$ were compared with the corresponding observed values to evaluate the accuracy of the model predictions. The results showed a slight underprediction of drug concentrations in children, with no bias in the case of term neonates and a bias towards overprediction in premature neonates. The premature neonates were not included in the detailed evaluation of the PK parameters; however, the model prediction overestimated clearance in term neonates who were a few days old. There was a bias toward overprediction of the predicted elimination $t_{1/2}$ in term neonates and children up to 18 years of age, whereas the V_d was adequately predicted for all children from birth to adolescence.

In 2011, Parrott et al. developed a model to simulate the PK of the orally administered drug oseltamivir and its active metabolite using the specialized modelling software Gastroplus® [23]. Although little experimental data were used, the results of the model evaluation showed an overprediction of drug exposure in neonates, with a >2-fold difference between the observed and predicted values and a trend towards higher deviation of model predictions in newborns when compared with infants.

Finally, while the publication by Johnson et al. [14] as well as the models reported by Kersting et al. [21] and Maharaj et al. [22] predicted the PK of intravenous etoposide and lorazepam in children of different ages, they did not include any neonatal data in the model evaluations.

As seen above, there are generally very few evaluated paediatric PBPK models and even fewer models incorporating neonatal data. On the one hand, this finding clearly highlights the need to report additional evaluated paediatric models, while on the other hand, it explains the uncertainties regarding the robustness and reliability of paediatric PBPK model predictions, especially after oral application, that persist in the paediatric community [24]. Only by showing the ability of such models to accurately replicate neonatal experimental data in humans can we close the gap between the theoretically immense potential applications of these models and the degree of confidence in the accuracy of the predictions they generate. The implementation of such techniques can then be further extended, especially to neonates, which is the age group that could benefit the most from robust models. An additional aspect to consider, whenever possible, is the stratification of the results by age group in future models, which could help detect any mechanisms or processes that are inadequately described in the model and could point to areas suitable for further research.

In addition, the previously mentioned examples show that the predictability of the models is relatively lower in neonates when compared to older children or adults. This can be explained, in part, by the rapid changes in the physiology and ontogeny of processes influencing drug disposition and by the high inter- and intra-individual variability in this population, which is influenced by multiple factors such as postgestational age or birth weight [25]. However, even with this comparatively higher error in neonates, it should be noted that the clinical relevance is always eventually judged by also taking into consideration the intended use of the model data and the allowable error for the drug, which is low for drugs with narrow therapeutic windows. For example, a deviation of more than a factor of 2 in predictions of a model in neonates may still be acceptable if the model-generated information will be used to suggest the sampling times in a future study whose aim is to perform an optimal PK analysis. However, the same error would be less acceptable or even unacceptable if the model were intended to be used to generate dosing recommendations for a substance with a narrow therapeutic window. In the latter case, any recommendations in neonates based on, for example, low predicted AUC values in comparison to the observed AUC could lead to a recommendation of higher therapeutic doses than necessary, with toxicity potentially likely to be an unintended clinical consequence.

Conclusion

In conclusion, PBPK models have immense potential to contribute to paediatric clinical trials and research, especially in neonates, where little or no available experimental data are available. The data provided by such models may help clinical trials become more 'confirmatory' rather than 'exploratory', saving time and effort and potentially reducing the number of children who need to be included. However, due to the current shortage of reported validated paediatric models in neonates, this exciting and promising technique still lacks the required evidence demonstrating that predictions generated by it are associated with error rates that are still acceptable for clinical use and that the predictions are as good in practice as they are in theory. Nevertheless, even with the current situation, it should be noted that both the purpose of the developed model as well as the type of the modelled drug play a major role in judging the suitability of employing model-generated predictions. Reporting more examples will help increase the degree of confidence in this technique and will definitely contribute to the wider implementation of PBPK modelling in paediatric research.

References

1 Bellanti F, Della Pasqua O: Modelling and simulation as research tools in paediatric drug development. Eur J Clin Pharmacol 2011;67(suppl 1):75–86.

2 Manolis E, Pons G: Proposals for model-based paediatric medicinal development within the current European Union regulatory framework. Br J Clin Pharmacol 2009;68:493–501.

3 Rowland M, Peck C, Tucker G: Physiologically-based pharmacokinetics in drug development and regulatory science. Annu Rev Pharmacol Toxicol 2011;51:45–73.

4 Manolis E, Osman TE, Herold R, Koenig F, Tomasi P, Vamvakas S, Saint Raymond A: Role of modeling and simulation in pediatric investigation plans. Paediatr Anaesth 2011;21:214–221.

5 Khalil F, Läer S: Physiologically based pharmacokinetic modeling: methodology, applications, and limitations with a focus on its role in pediatric drug development. J Biomed Biotechnol 2011;2011:907461.

6 Commission of the European Communities: Regulation (EC) No 1901/2006 of the European Parliament and of the council of 12 December 2006 on medicinal products for paediatric use and amending Regulation (EEC) No 1768/92, Directive 2001/20/EC, Directive 2001/83/EC and Regulation (EC) No 726/2004. Official Journal of the European Union 2006;L378:1–19.

7 International Conference on Harmonisation: Guidance on E11 clinical investigation of medicinal products in the pediatric population; availability. Notice. Fed Regist 2000;65:78493–78494.

8 Nestorov I: Whole body pharmacokinetic models. Clin Pharmacokinet 2003;42:883–908.

9 Willmann S, Lippert J, Sevestre M, Solodenko J, Fois F, Schmitt W: PK-Sim®: a physiologically based pharmacokinetic 'whole-body' model. Biosilico 2003;1:121–124.

10 Jamei M, Marciniak S, Feng K, Barnett A, Tucker G, Rostami-Hodjegan A: The Simcyp population-based ADME simulator. Expert Opin Drug Metab Toxicol 2009;5:211–223.

11 Hsien L: Identifying Paediatric Needs in Cardiology and the Prediction of Sildenafil Exposure in Children with Pulmonary Arterial Hypertension. Thesis. Düsseldorf, University of Düsseldorf, 2010.

12 Willmann S: The in silico child. Can computer simulations replace clinical pharmacokinetic studies? Pharm Unserer Zeit 2009;38:62–67.

13 Dumont C, Mentre F, Gaynor C, Brendel K, Gesson C, Chenel M: Optimal sampling times for a drug and its metabolite using SIMCYP® simulations as prior information. Clin Pharmacokinet 2013;52:43–57.

14 Johnson TN, Rostami-Hodjegan A: Resurgence in the use of physiologically based pharmacokinetic models in pediatric clinical pharmacology: parallel shift in incorporating the knowledge of biological elements and increased applicability to drug development and clinical practice. Paediatr Anaesth 2011; 21:291–301.
15 Edginton AN, Ritter L: Predicting plasma concentrations of bisphenol A in children younger than 2 years of age after typical feeding schedules, using a physiologically based toxicokinetic model. Environ Health Perspect 2009;117:645–652.
16 Johnson TN, Rostami-Hodjegan A, Tucker GT: Prediction of the clearance of eleven drugs and associated variability in neonates, infants and children. Clin Pharmacokinet 2006;45:931–956.
17 Edginton AN, Schmitt W, Voith B, Willmann S: A mechanistic approach for the scaling of clearance in children. Clin Pharmacokinet 2006;45:683–704.
18 Ginsberg G, Hattis D, Russ A, Sonawane B: Physiologically based pharmacokinetic (PBPK) modeling of caffeine and theophylline in neonates and adults: implications for assessing children's risks from environmental agents. J Toxicol Environ Health A 2004; 67:297–329.
19 Björkman S: Prediction of drug disposition in infants and children by means of physiologically based pharmacokinetic (PBPK) modelling: theophylline and midazolam as model drugs. Br J Clin Pharmacol 2005;59:691–704.
20 Edginton AN, Schmitt W, Willmann S: Development and evaluation of a generic physiologically based pharmacokinetic model for children. Clin Pharmacokinet 2006;45:1013–1034.
21 Kersting G, Willmann S, Wurthwein G, Lippert J, Boos J, Hempel G: Physiologically based pharmacokinetic modelling of high- and low-dose etoposide: from adults to children. Cancer Chemother Pharmacol 2012;69:397–405.
22 Maharaj AR, Barrett JS, Edginton AN: A workflow example of PBPK modeling to support pediatric research and development: case study with lorazepam. AAPS J 2013;15:455–464.
23 Parrott N, Davies B, Hoffmann G, Koerner A, Lave T, Prinssen E, Theogaraj E, Singer T: Development of a physiologically based model for oseltamivir and simulation of pharmacokinetics in neonates and infants. Clin Pharmacokinet 2011;50:613–623.
24 Barrett JS, Della Casa Alberighi O, Läer S, Meibohm B: Physiologically based pharmacokinetic (PBPK) modeling in children. Clin Pharmacol Ther 2012;92: 40–49.
25 Tayman C, Rayyan M, Allegaert K: Neonatal pharmacology: extensive interindividual variability despite limited size. J Pediatr Pharmacol Ther 2011;16: 170–184.

Stephanie Läer
Institute of Clinical Pharmacy and Pharmacotherapy
Heinrich-Heine University of Düsseldorf, Universitätsstrasse 1, Geb. 26.22.02.21
DE–40225 Düsseldorf (Germany)
E-Mail stephanie.laeer@uni-duesseldorf.de

Mimouni FB, van den Anker JN (eds): Neonatal Pharmacology and Nutrition Update.
Pediatr Adolesc Med. Basel, Karger, 2015, vol 18, pp 70–82 (DOI: 10.1159/000365029)

A Systematic Review of Paracetamol and Closure of Patent Ductus Arteriosus: Ready for Prime Time?

Cathy Hammerman[a, b] · Francis B. Mimouni[a, c] · Alona Bin-Nun[a]

[a]Department of Neonatology, Shaare Zedek Medical Center, Jerusalem, [b]Hebrew University, Faculty of Medicine, Jerusalem, and [c]Tel Aviv University, Sackler School of Medicine, Tel Aviv, Israel

Abstract

Over the past decade, the neonatal literature has undergone dynamic swings vis a vis its approach to patent ductus arteriosus (PDA) therapeutics, from aggressively closing all PDA's to permissive tolerance of ductal shunting. We propose that ductal closure with paracetamol can satisfy both sides of this debate by offering a non-invasive therapeutic option with minimal potential toxicity. We review all of the available clinical experience with paracetamol and the ductus, as well as its potential for toxicity.

In medicine, we are constantly exhorted to remember the directive *primum non nocere*. While refraining from harming our patients is a worthy principle in guiding therapeutic interventions, its implementation can, at times, become unexpectedly confusing. The therapeutic approach to patent ductus arteriosus (PDA) in the preterm neonate demonstrates just such a clinical conundrum. Over the past decade, the neonatal literature has undergone dynamic swings, vis a vis its approach to PDA therapeutics, such that it is often hard to define what is best for our patients.

We have been increasingly urged to adopt a 'kinder, gentler approach' to persistent PDA, encouraging a permissive tolerance of ductal shunting while awaiting spontaneous closure and withholding therapy in all except the most hemodynamically significant cases [1–8]. This approach has been advocated based on the lack of convincing evidence to support the once common practice of early aggressive pharmacologic closure coupled with the serious side effects of COX inhibitors. These include altered platelet function, decreased cerebral, mesenteric and renal blood flow resulting in altered renal function, and gastrointestinal perforation, which although mostly reversible, can occasionally be clinically challenging and, in some cases, even life-threatening [9, 10].

However, lack of evidence is not the same as evidence of a lack of effect. While the kinder, gentler approach has led to a significant reduction in both the therapeutic and prophylactic administration of indomethacin and ibuprofen, data are again beginning to emerge suggesting increased long-term morbidities that are possibly associated with or exacerbated by not treating a PDA.

Recent studies have associated increased morbidity and mortality with both the presence of an early PDA [11] and with a persistent patent ductus that has failed to close [12]. Nevertheless, association does not prove causation and hence still does not offer a definitive mandate for therapeutic intervention. There is, however, one recent, large retrospective review [13] that does provide evidence-based support for re-evaluating our approach to treat a PDA. This review compares long-term outcomes of two different ductal treatments in Vermont Oxford Network centers, and it documents surprising increases in chronic lung disease when PDA's were treated with 'permissive tolerance'. As a result, the pendulum of public opinion is again shifting as we realize that permissive tolerance may have actually evolved into a form of benign neglect.

Thus, it is possible that closing the patent ductus is still hemodynamically beneficial for many infants and that an alternative treatment with fewer potential side effects might be helpful in resolving some of the therapeutic dilemmas. Paracetamol (also named acetaminophen), the latest addition to the therapeutic arsenal against PDA [14] might offer just such a therapeutic alternative. As such, we feel that it is important, at this time, to review the current status of the relevant paracetamol literature as it relates to ductal closure.

We, therefore, performed a systematic review of all cases reported in the literature. Searches were performed using Medline, Google Scholar, and Embase. A standard search strategy for paracetamol and PDA was implemented. A second search, including paracetamol/acetaminophen and toxicity, overdose (age) or hepatotoxicity, was executed, and all references were analyzed. The authors were contacted for clarification when data were unclear or undefined, and in one case, this resulted in an expanded study population. The data from this personal communication were included in our subsequent analysis.

Observational Studies

In 2011, we published the first series of case reports [14] documenting the efficacy of paracetamol in mediating ductal closure in five premature neonates with hemodynamically significant PDAs. Since 2011, 10 additional observational series have been published, collectively treating a total of 80 infants with an overall ductal closure rate

Table 1. Observational studies

	Study population – description	Route of drug administration	Birth weight*, g	Gestational age*, weeks	Post-natal age*, DOL	Outcome (% PDA closure)	Elevated transaminases
Hammerman et al. [14] (n = 5)	Ibuprofen failure (n = 3) or contraindication (n = 2)	Enteral	935 [851–1,053]	27.2±1.6	10 [8–21]	5/5 (100)	0
Oncel et al. [15] (n = 8)	Ibuprofen failure (n = 5) or contraindication (n = 2)	Enteral	995 [630–2,970]	28.5 [24–37]	9.5 [5–27]	7/8 (87.5)	0
Yurttutan et al. [16] (n = 6)	First-line drug	Enteral	1,260 [920–1,600]	28.5 [26–32]	5.5 [3–7]	5/6 (83)	0
Oncel et al. [17] (n = 10)	First-line drug	Intravenous	775 [590–990]	24.6 [24–29]	6 [2–15]	10/10 (100)	0
Tekgunduz et al. [18] (n = 7)	First-line drug	Intravenous	1,104 [770–1,390]	29.3 [27–31]	5.0 [2–9]	6/7 (86)	1 elevated transaminase at 15-mg dose. Drug stopped, and transaminases returned to normal
Alan et al. [19] (n = 3)	All ibuprofen failures	Intravenous	963 [810–1,240]	28.6 [26.2–33.5]	12.0 [8–19]	0/3 (0)	2/3 – transiently elevated transaminases
Sinha et al. [21] (n = 10)	First-line drug	Enteral	1,052 [800–1,380]	29.5 [27–33]	4.9 [4–7]	10/10 (100)	0
Jasani et al. [22] (n = 6)	Ibuprofen failure (n = 4) or contraindication (n = 2)	Enteral	1,115 [1,040–1,235]	29.9 [28.6–31.1]	5.6 [3–9]	6/6 (100)	0
Ozdemir et al. [23] *Need for clinical trials in neonates* (n = 7)	All ibuprofen failures	Enteral	936	26	36.2±11.6	5/7 (71.4)	0
Terrin et al. [25] (n = 8)	First-line drug	Intravenous	724±173	26±2	2.8±1.2	6/8 (75)	0
Roofthooft et al. [20] (n = 10)	Ibuprofen failure (n = 6) or contraindication (n = 4) 8 patients received ibuprofen	Intravenous (n = 9) Enteral (n = 1)	700 [365–950]	25±1	22.0 [13–30]	2/10 (20)	0
Nadir et al. [26] (n = 7)	Ibuprofen contraindicated (n = 7)	Enteral	656–2,415	24–27	10.5±7.7	5/7 (71)	0

* Data are presented as the median [interquartile range] or mean ± standard deviation, depending on how the data were presented by the individual authors.

of above 85% [15–24] (table 1). This degree of therapeutic efficacy compares favorably with that achieved by standard therapy with cyclo-oxygenase inhibitors, which is generally quoted to be around 70% [24], and this is a necessary although not sufficient factor in achieving widespread acceptance of any new therapy.

Paracetamol owes its rapidly growing popularity to several additional factors. As one of most commonly used over-the-counter drugs worldwide, it offers familiarity, availability and financial feasibility. Furthermore, it presents certain practical as well as theoretical advantages over both ibuprofen and indomethacin, including the potential to treat those with contraindications to the use of COX inhibitors and the absence of any known peripheral vasoconstrictive effects. In fact, at the administered doses, paracetamol has minimal known toxicity.

Effect of Prior Exposure to Ibuprofen

Most of the infants treated with paracetamol in the observational studies either had contraindications to ibuprofen therapy, and paracetamol was given as initial treatment for PDA closure, or previous attempts at closure with ibuprofen had failed, and paracetamol was given as a second, rescue therapy. When these two groups were analyzed separately, a clear advantage to treating with paracetamol as a first-line drug became evident. In five of the series, paracetamol was predominantly given solely as a first-line drug to infants with contraindications to ibuprofen. In total, we have identified 55 neonates who were not pre-exposed to ibuprofen. This includes infants from the above-mentioned first-line-drug studies, infants from studies with mixed-entry criteria who were not given ibuprofen because of contraindications and additional infants from an expansion of the Roofthooft study (personal communication from S. Simons). The PDAs of 49 of these 55 infants (89%) closed with paracetamol, compared with 16 of 36 PDAs (44%) in infants in whom paracetamol was given as a second-line drug ($p < 0.001$).

Effect of Postnatal Age

It is possible that those treated following ibuprofen failures were merely treated at a later postnatal age and that it is early treatment, as suggested by Terrin et al. [25], that actually accounts for the therapeutic advantage. In fact, earlier treatment does appear to be associated with improved responsiveness. The two studies with the highest failure rates [19, 20] began paracetamol treatment 12 and 22 days postnatally. However, the Ozdemir study [23] initiated treatment at 36 days of age and had a 71% success rate. From the data as it is published (means or medians), it is impossible to ascertain the age of treatment for specific cases of failed response, thereby precluding more precise statistical analysis.

Effect of the Route of Administration

Five of the studies administered their paracetamol intravenously, while the remaining five used an enteral solution. Although the overwhelming majority of both groups showed good efficacy, there were differences between these two routes of administration, with a clear favoring toward enteral administration. Ductal closure was achieved in 94% of those treated enterally vs. 68% of those treated intravenously (p = 0.01), an interesting observation, although somewhat counterintuitive, and deserving of further study. Interestingly, in this context, similar data show that enteral ibuprofen may be more effective than parenteral ibuprofen (84.6 vs. 62% PDA closure rate; p = 0.011) [27]. In that study, the authors hypothesized that absorption was slower with oral ibuprofen than with intravenous ibuprofen, thereby prolonging the time of contact with the ductus and leading to a higher response rate.

Furthermore, of all 80 patients collectively reported in these observational studies, there were three patients who showed mildly and transiently elevated liver enzymes. These three were treated intravenously. There were no elevated transaminases observed in any infants treated with enteral paracetamol. While the numbers are too small to draw any statistically valid conclusions, there may be cause for concern here, and this observation clearly warrants further examination in future studies.

Dosing

All of the reported studies except for one used paracetamol (both enteral and intravenous) at a dose of 15 mg/kg/dose (60 mg/kg/day). Only one study looked at the effect of a reduced paracetamol dose. Tekgunduz et al. [18] began treating patients with doses of 15 mg/kg every six hours in their study using intravenous paracetamol. However, after 4 doses, they noted significant increases in transaminase levels in their first infant compared to pretreatment concentrations (AST 260 vs. 43 U/l; ALT 180 vs. 11 U/l). The drug was stopped, and the transaminase concentrations normalized over the following 4 days. After this experience, they decreased both the individual doses as well as the dosing interval (to 30 mg/kg/day), and they reported closure of all ducts when the infant was treated with this new approach. Arana et al. [28] have suggested an oral-dosing schedule for small premature infants consisting of a 20-mg/kg loading dose followed by a maintenance dose of 15 mg/kg/dose given every 12 h. However, it must be remembered that these recommendations are based on data regarding pain and temperature regulation and that we have no indication as to the optimal dosing for ductal closure.

Pharmacokinetics and Safety: Minimal Potential Hepatotoxicity

Safety concerns regarding paracetamol dosing have been raised by Allegaert et al. [29]. Of note, these concerns primarily rely upon pharmacokinetic calculations based on data derived from intravenous paracetamol administration given to more mature neonates. There is a paucity of relevant actual safety data on enteral administration in preterm neonates.

Anderson et al. [30] pooled data from six separate neonatal pharmacokinetic studies. They describe a target concentration of 10 mg/ml as the steady state concentration that is reported to be effective for both temperature reduction and pain management. However, we are unaware of what paracetamol concentrations to aim for vis a vis the induction of ductal closure.

Only two of the observational PDA studies measured serum paracetamol concentrations. Oncel et al. [17] measured serum levels on days 1 (7.3 mcg/ml), 2 (15.5 mcg/ml) and 3 (14.7 mcg/ml) of intravenous paracetamol treatment, while in the study by Yurttutan et al. [16] serum paracetamol levels were evaluated 24 h after the first dose of enteral paracetamol, and the levels ranged from 5 to 18 mcg/ml. The values from both studies are well within the normal range of 10–30 mcg/ml for children [31] and far from those causing any concern of toxicity in term neonates and older children.

Theoretical pharmacokinetic concerns notwithstanding, the major worry regarding the clinical level is the possibility of hepatotoxicity. More than 90% of acetaminophen is metabolized in the liver via two conjugation pathways – glucuronidation and sulfation – and the remainder is oxidized by the cytochrome P-450 CYP2E1 mixed-function oxidase system, which is composed of 3 isoforms, CYP2E1, CYP3A4, and CYP1A2. The product of this oxidation is the toxic metabolite (N-acetyl-p-benzoquinone imine [NAPQI]) that is then rapidly detoxified by glutathione and eliminated in urine or bile. However, when paracetamol is taken in excess, the body's glutathione reserves become insufficient to inactivate NAPQI. NAPQI that has not been detoxified accumulates and is then free to bind to hepatocytes, leading to hepatic necrosis and failure [30].

Furthermore, any concurrent administration of a drug that induces the cytochrome system may increase the amount of NAPQI produced, thus increasing the likelihood of acetaminophen toxicity. Binding of NAPQI to cysteine groups on hepatocyte proteins forms acetaminophen-protein adducts that may be released into the serum and have been correlated with liver injury in animal models. Although they can also be found in 10% of children with acute liver failure not associated with acetaminophen [32], they may prove to be helpful indicators of occult hepatotoxicity in future prospective clinical studies [33].

Overall, however, neonatal toxicity is low. Neonates have relatively low levels of CYP2E1 enzyme activity, thereby slowing oxidative metabolism of paracetamol in the neonate and reducing the production of toxic metabolites. Neonates also have an increased rate of glutathione synthesis. This combination in preterm infants presumably confers some level of protective benefit in the event of an overdose [34].

The reported clinical experiences with paracetamol overdoses in infants support the theoretical lower toxicity. Table 2 summarizes all of the 10 reported cases of neonates exposed to potentially toxic amounts of paracetamol that our searches revealed [35–42]. The long-term outcomes were universally favorable, despite transient elevations in liver enzymes being reported in half of the cases. To the best of our knowledge, there are no cases in the literature describing permanent liver damage secondary to

Table 2. Reported cases of paracetamol overdose in neonates

	Clinical details of overdose	GA, weeks	Postnatal age (DOL)	Treatment	Peak measured serum paracetamol concentration	Outcome
Porta et al. [33]	436 mg/kg IV	25.5	12	N-acetyl-cysteine	180 mcg/ml 5 h after discovery of the overdose	No increase in liver enzymes, bilirubin, or prothrombin time
Isbister et al. [35]	136 mg/kg oral paracetamol (received 300 mg instead of 30 mg)	29	55	Naso-gastric charcoal	121 mcg/ml four hours after ingestion	No hepatotoxicity
Nolent et al. [36]	Accidentally given an intramuscular injection of 211 mg/kg propacetamol (equivalent to 105.5 mg/kg paracetamol) on the first day of life	41	1	N-acetyl-cysteine		Liver enzymes remained normal during hospitalization and after discharge
Nevin et al. [37]	380 mg of intravenous paracetamol (146 mg/kg) was inadvertently administered during anesthesia	28	7 weeks	N-acetyl-cysteine	117 mcg/ml 4 h after ingestion	
Brener et al. [38]	266 mg/kg in three doses	27	9	N-acetyl-cysteine	480 mcg/ml	No elevation of liver enzymes
Walls et al. [39]	Oral acetaminophen after circumcision; 80 mg (26 mg/kg) every 4 h for the first 24 h (156 mg/kg/day), then 40 mg every 4 h for the next 2 days (78 mg/kg/day)	41	13	N-acetyl-cysteine	109.8 mcg/ml 16 h after last dose	AST 718 mg/l upon admission. Improved over several days, and he became more alert. No residual effects
De la Pintière et al. [40]	Following a prescribing error, a female term newborn was given two intravenous doses of 900 mg propacetamol (307 mg/kg/dose) mg/kg IV at 6-h intervals	40	First days of life	N-acetyl-cysteine	168 mcg/ml	No hepatotoxicity
Muniz et al. [41]	Multiple administrations of 80 mg (16.32 mg/kg/dose) 97.9 mg/kg/day	40	58	N-acetyl-cysteine	287 mcg/ml	Admitted with elevated liver enzymes, which peaked on day 3. Complete resolution of all clinical and laboratory abnormalities upon follow-up
Pham et al. [42]	400 mg of acetaminophen at 6-h intervals (157 mg/kg per dose); total dose of 845 mg of acetaminophen over 17 h	40	First days of life	N-acetyl-cysteine	173 mcg/ml	No hepatotoxicity and clinically no long-term sequelae
Brener et al. [38]	Received three doses at 266 mg/kg	27	9	N-acetyl-cysteine	480 mcg/ml	No short- or long-term clinical symptoms

paracetamol poisoning in a newborn by directly administering the drug to a neonate, although extra caution needs to be exercised in cases in which there is pre-existing liver damage from other causes.

Within the 80 patients described to date in the observational paracetamol PDA case reports, there were three infants with transiently elevated liver transaminases. All three were treated with intravenous paracetamol. Of interest is the fact that, in these three cases, paracetamol treatment failed to close the ductus. The rate of hepatotoxicity is thus significantly higher in the treatment failures compared with the successes (15.8 vs. 0.0%, p = 0.002), despite the fact that the doses were similar. It should be noted that in one of the cases [18], treatment was stopped after four doses when it was noted that transaminases were increased. This tendency for hepatotoxicity to occur primarily in subjects in whom the duct fails to close raises speculation vis a vis the possibility of some early metabolic diversion towards the oxidative NAPQI pathway in these infants. These observations warrant further investigation in future studies.

Pharmacokinetics and Safety: Asthma Association

In 1998, Varner et al. first suggested that the rising prevalence of asthma might be related to the declining use of aspirin in favor of increasing exposure to paracetamol [43]. Since then, many articles have been published attempting to relate early paracetamol consumption to the development of asthma. The data presented below are not intended to present a comprehensive review of these many studies, but rather a representative sampling that highlights some of the strengths and weaknesses of these data. In an analysis of a large sample of children and adolescents included in the International Study of Asthma and Allergies in Childhood (ISAAC), Beasley et al. observed a relationship between paracetamol ingestion in the first year of life and symptoms of asthma, rhinitis and eczema at 6–7 years of age [44]. Similar observations were reported in a birth-cohort study from New Zealand that suggested a link between paracetamol exposure before the age of 15 months and atopy at 6 years; however, this group was not able to document a significant effect on asthma [45]. Rusconi et al. [46] found that administration of paracetamol and antibiotics during the first year of life was associated with early wheezing, whereas the association between paracetamol and late-onset wheezing was not significant. Lowe et al. prospectively studied 620 children with family histories of allergic disease. In their study, children who took paracetamol for non-respiratory illnesses showed no increased risk of asthma [47].

In summary, this brief sampling shows that the relevant studies suffer from substantial methodological problems, ranging from significant heterogeneity in study outcome (early wheezing vs. late wheezing vs. atopy) to the lack of adjustment for confounding variables, yielding contradictory results. The overwhelming majority of these studies are of a retrospective design, relying on maternal recall of paracetamol administration in infancy correlated with subsequent asthma symptoms, rather than being specifically designed as prospective, randomized studies powered to determine whether paracetamol actually causes asthma.

At best, these studies demonstrate an association, and no causal relationship has been established. In fact, because the presence of recurrent respiratory tract infections is likely to be a determining factor in both asthma development and in increased paracetamol usage, it is entirely possible that paracetamol may merely be an

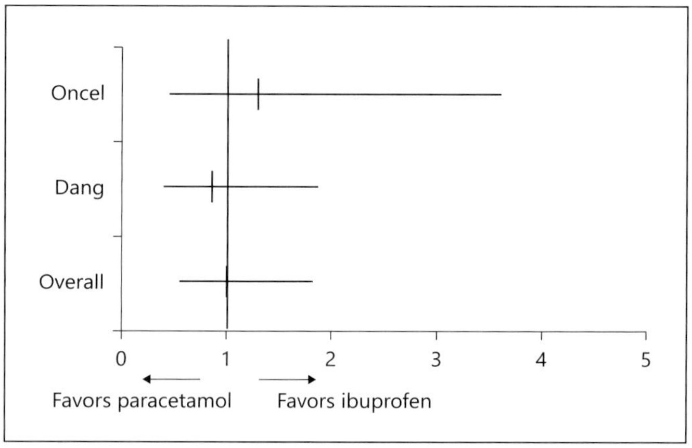

Fig. 1. PDA closure rate. Forest plot of the meta-analysis of the two randomized controlled trials showing no difference in PDA closure rates in either an individual trial or overall.

innocent bystander in this complex process. This idea is supported by the Rusconi study [46], which looked at correlations between antibiotic and paracetamol usage and early wheezing. Although they found both to be associated, the correlation between antibiotic usage and early wheezing was stronger than that between paracetamol and wheezing.

Nevertheless, the possibility of a causal relationship, albeit unproven, should be taken into consideration when weighing the pros and cons of choosing paracetamol for ductal closure.

Randomized Controlled Studies

In the recent months, two prospective, randomized trials comparing the efficacy of paracetamol with that of ibuprofen in mediating ductal closure have been published [48, 49]. Both ibuprofen and paracetamol were administered enterally with similar protocols in both studies, and paracetamol was given at a dose of 15 mg/kg every 6 h for 3 days. Together, the two studies included 240 infants. Figures 1 and 2 present a meta-analysis of the PDA response data from both studies that confirms that, overall, the rates of PDA closure and PDA recurrences were similar between those treated with paracetamol and ibuprofen.

These studies were powered to detect a 20–25% difference in the ductal closure rate between the two drugs, which they did not find. Overall, both studies concluded that paracetamol, when used as a first-line drug, had an efficacy similar to that of ibuprofen in mediating ductal closure. In the Oncel study [48], a secondary analysis was done on gestational age subgroups. When infants ≤26 weeks were considered independently, there was a trend towards improved closure (56.2 vs. 76.9%) in the paracetamol group that did not reach significance, as the numbers within each of the subgroups were quite small. There were 16 infants in the ibuprofen group and 13 infants in the

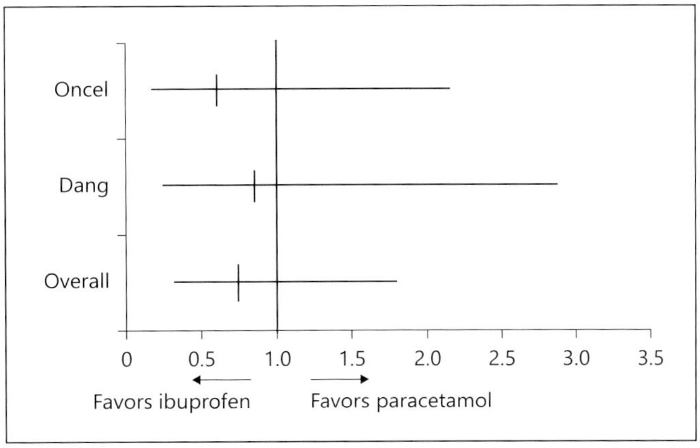

Fig. 2. PDA recurrence rate. Forest plot of the meta-analysis of the two randomized controlled trials showing no difference in PDA recurrence rates in either an individual trial or overall.

paracetamol subgroup, while a sample size of 81 infants in each group would have been needed to reach a significance of $p < 0.05$ with a power of 80% with this degree of difference in the response rate. In the Dang study [49], significant reductions in hyperbilirubinemia (20 vs. 35%; $p = 0.03$) and in gastrointestinal bleeding (2.5 vs. 10%; $p = 0.03$) were noted in the paracetamol group compared with the ibuprofen-treated infants. Other specific parameters, such as the route of administration and prior exposure to COX inhibitors, noted to be of potential significance in the observational studies, cannot be evaluated within the context of the randomized control studies because the protocols precluded differences in these areas.

There was no reported evidence of hepatotoxicity in either group of either study. There was a trend, albeit not significant, toward a higher incidence of retinopathy of prematurity (ROP) in ibuprofen-treated groups in both studies. Although the literature on COX inhibitors and ROP appears to be contradictory on the surface, we postulated [50] re-interpreting these data within the context of the biphasic paradigm of ROP pathophysiology. As in these studies, drugs with a vasoconstrictive effect may potentially exacerbate ROP when given during the initial hyperoxic phase of the process, while they may have an opposite effect if given later on. Thus, the trend towards increased ROP may reflect the early ibuprofen treatment in these trials.

In summary, the prospective, randomized trials show that paracetamol and ibuprofen have similar overall efficacy. Although a trend towards improved closure was evident in the smallest infants, the studies were not sufficiently powered to confirm this. The observational case reports point to enteral administration at an earlier postnatal age, with no prior exposure to ibuprofen, in order to obtain the best chance of therapeutic success. Further studies are clearly needed to resolve issues such as optimal dosing levels and dose-concentration-effect studies; and randomized studies using new techniques such as metabolomics will be important in defining and/or excluding any potential major issues, such as the possibility of an increased risk of asthma that is secondary to exposure to paracetamol. However, these basic questions notwithstanding, we believe that the concerns must be evaluated in relation to the currently accepted drugs used for PDA closure. Both ibuprofen and indomethacin are associated with safety concerns of their own, which are no less troubling than the hypothetical concerns raised regarding paracetamol administration. We therefore believe that the existing data are sufficient to support consideration by the FDA of paracetamol as one of the therapeutic options in the pharmacologic approach to hemodynamically significant PDA in the premature neonate. For the purpose of comparison, it is worth pointing out that the FDA awarded approval for the use of ibuprofen for PDA closure, despite its potential side effects, based on a study that included only 136 infants [51], which was less than the 240 infants who have already taken part in the prospective paracetamol trials.

References

1 Bose CL, Laughon MM: Patent ductus arteriosus: lack of evidence for common treatments. Arch Dis Child Fetal Neonatal Ed 2007;92:F498–F502.

2 Benitz WE: Treatment of persistent patent ductus arteriosus in preterm infants: time to accept the null hypothesis? J Perinatol 2010;30:241–252.

3 Benitz WE: Patent ductus arteriosus: to treat or not to treat? Arch Dis Child Fetal Neonatal Ed 2012; 97:F80–F82.

4 Laughon MM, Simmons MA, Bose CL: Patency of the ductus arteriosus in the premature infant: is it pathologic? Should it be treated? Curr Opin Pediatr 2004;16:146–151.

5 Fowlie PW: Managing the baby with a patent ductus arteriosus. More questions than answers? Arch Dis Child Fetal Neonatal Ed 2005;90:F190.

6 Schmidt B, Davis P, Moddemann D, Ohlsson A, Roberts RS, Saigal S, et al: Long-term effects of indomethacin prophylaxis in extremely-low-birth-weight infants. N Engl J Med 2001;344:1966–1972.

7 Clyman RI, Chorne N: Patent ductus arteriosus: evidence for and against treatment. J Pediatr 2007;150: 216–219.

8 Van Overmeire B: Patent ductus arteriosus: how aggressive should we be? Neonatology 2007;91:318.

9 Paquette L, Friedlich P, Ramanathan R, Seri I: Concurrent use of indomethacin and dexamethasone increases the risk of spontaneous intestinal perforation in very low birth weight neonates. J Perinatol 2006; 26:486–492.

10 Gournay V, Roze JC, Kuster A, Daoud P, Cambonie G, Hascoet JM, et al: Prophylactic ibuprofen versus placebo in very premature infants: a randomized, double-blind, placebo-controlled trial. Lancet 2004; 364:1939–1944.

11 Sellmer A, Vandborg Bjerre J, Schmidt M, McNamara P, Hjortdal V, Host B, et al: Morbidity and mortality in preterm neonates with patent ductus arteriosus on day 3. Arch Dis Child Fetal Neonatal Ed 2013;98:F505–F510.

12 Noori S, McCoy M, Friedlich P, Bright B, Gottipati V, Seri I, et al: Failure of ductus arteriosus closure is associated with increased mortality in preterm neonates. Pediatrics 2009;123:e138–e144.

13 Kaempf JW, Huston R, Wu YX, Kaempf AJ, Wang L, Grunkemeier G, et al: Permissive tolerance of the patent ductus arteriosus may increase the risk of chronic lung disease. Research and Reports in Neonatology 2013;3:5–10.

14 Hammerman C, Bin-Nun A, Markovitch E, Schimmel MS: Ductal closure with paracetamol: a surprising new approach to patent ductus arteriosus treatment. Pediatrics 2011;128:e1–e4.

15 Oncel MY, Yurttutan S, Uras N, Altug N, Ozdemir R, Ekmen S, et al: An alternative drug (paracetamol) in the management of patent ductus arteriosus in ibuprofen-resistant or contraindicated preterm infants. Arch Dis Child Fetal Neonatal Ed 2013;98:F94.

16 Yurttutan S, Oncel MY, Arayıcı S, Uras N, Altug N, Erdeve O, et al: A different first-choice drug in the medical management of patent ductus arteriosus: oral paracetamol. J Matern Fetal Neonatal Med 2013; 26:825–827.

17 Oncel MY, Yurttutan S, Degirmencioglu H, Uras N, Altug N, Erdeve O, et al: Intravenous paracetamol treatment in the management of patent ductus arteriosus in extremely low birth weight infants. Neonatology 2013;103:166–169.

18 Tekgunduz KS, Ceviz N, Demirelli Y, Olgun H, Caner I, Sahin IO, et al: Intravenous paracetamol for patent ductus arteriosus in premature infants – a lower dose is also effective. Neonatology 2013;104:6–7.

19 Alan S, Kahvecioglu D, Erdeve O, Atasay B, Arsan S: Is paracetamol a useful treatment for ibuprofen-resistant patent ductus arteriosus? Neonatology 2013;104:168–169.
20 Roofthooft DW, van Beynum IM, Helbing WA, Reiss IK, Simons SH: Paracetamol for ductus arteriosus closure: not always a success story. Neonatology 2013;104:170.
21 Sinha R, Negi V, Dalal SS: An interesting observation of PDA closure with oral paracetamol in preterm neonates. J Clin Neonatol 2013;2:30–32.
22 Jasani B, Kabra N, Nanavati RN: Oral paracetamol in treatment of closure of patent ductus arteriosus in preterm neonates. J Postgrad Med 2013;59:312–314.
23 Ozdemir OM, Doğan M, Küçüktaşçı K, Ergin H, Sahin O: Paracetamol therapy for patent ductus arteriosus in premature infants: a chance before surgical ligation. Pediatr Cardiol 2014;35:276–279.
24 Ohlsson A, Walia R, Shah SS: Ibuprofen for the treatment of patent ductus arteriosus in preterm and/or low birth weight infants. Cochrane Database Syst Rev 2010;4:CD003481.
25 Terrin G, Conte F, Scipione A, Oncel MY, Simons SHP, Sinha R, et al: Paracetamol for treatment of patent ductus arteriosus: a systematic review. [Submitted for publication].
26 Nadir E, Kassem E, Foldi S, Hochberg A, Feldman M: Paracetamol treatment of patent ductus arteriosus in preterm infants. J Perinatol 2014, DOI: 10.1038/jp.2014.96 (Epub ahead of print).
27 Gokmen T, Erdeve O, Altug N, Oguz SS, Uras N, Dilmen U: Efficacy and safety of oral versus intravenous ibuprofen in very low birth weight preterm infants with patent ductus arteriosus. J Pediatr 2011;158:549–554.
28 Arana A, Morton NS, Hansen TG: Treatment with paracetamol in infants. Acta Anaesthesiol Scand 2001;45:20–29.
29 Allegaert K, Anderson B, Simons S, van Overmeire B: Paracetamol to induce ductus arteriosus closure: Is it valid? Arch Dis Child 2013;98:462–466.
30 Anderson BJ, van Lingen R, Hansen TG, Lin YC, Holford NH: Acetaminophen developmental pharmacokinetics in premature neonates and infants: a pooled population analysis. Anesthesiology 2002;96:1336–1345.
31 Kratz A, Ferraro M, Sluss PM, Lewandrowski KB: Case records of the Massachusetts General Hospital: laboratory values. N Engl J Med 2004;351:1549–1563.
32 James LP, Wilson JT, Simar R, Farrar HC, Kearns GL, Simpson PM, et al: Evaluation of occult acetaminophen hepatotoxicity in hospitalized children receiving acetaminophen. Pediatric Pharmacology Research Unit Network. Clin Pediatr (Phila) 2001;40:243–248.
33 Porta R, Sánchez L, Nicolás M, García C, Martínez M: Lack of toxicity after paracetamol overdose in a extremely preterm neonate. Eur J Clin Pharmacol 2012;68:901–902.
34 James LP, Alonso EM, Hynan LS, Hinson JA, Davern TJ, Lee WM, et al: Detection of acetaminophen protein adducts in children with acute liver failure of indeterminate cause. Pediatrics 2006;118:e676–e681.
35 Isbister GK, Bucens IK, Whyte IM: Paracetamol overdose in a preterm neonate. Arch Dis Child Fetal Neonatal Ed 2001;85:F70–F72.
36 Nolent P: Intramuscular injection of propacetamol in a neonate. Arch Dis Child Fetal Neonatal Ed 2002;87:F155–F156.
37 Nevin DG, Shung J: Intravenous paracetamol overdose in a preterm infant during anesthesia. Paediatr Anaesth 2010;20:105–107.
38 Brener P, Ballardo M, Mariani G, Ceriani-Cernadas JM: Medication error in an extremely low birth weight infant: paracetamol overdose. Arch Argent Pediatr 2013;111:53–55.
39 Walls L, Baker CF, Sarkar S: Acetaminophen induced-hepatic failure with encephalopathy in a newborn. J Perinatol 2007;27:133–135.
40 De la Pintière A, Beuchée A, Bétrémieux PE: Intravenous paracetamol overdose in a term newborn. Arch Dis Child Fetal Neonatal Ed 2003;88:351–352.
41 Muniz AE, Rose SR 2nd, Liner SR, Foster RL: Unsuspected acetaminophen toxicity in a 58-day-old infant. Pediatr Emerg Care 2004;20:824–828.
42 Pham YT, Giraud C, Miossec E, Lejeune C, Callanquin M: Medicinal error during intravenous infusion with acetaminophen: Case of an overdose in neonatology. Journal de Pharmacie Clinique 2004;23:181–187.
43 Varner AE, Busse WW, Lemanske RF: Hypothesis: decreased use of pediatric aspirin has contributed to the increasing prevalence of childhood asthma. Ann Allergy Asthma Immunol 1998;81:347–351.
44 Beasley R, Clayton T, Crane J, von Mutis E, Lai CKW, Montefort S, et al: Association between paracetamol use in infancy and childhood, and risk of asthma, rhinoconjunctivitis, and eczema in children aged 6–7 years: analysis from Phase Three of the ISAAC programme. Lancet 2008;372:1039–1048.
45 Wickens K, Beasley R, Town I, Epton M, Pattemore P, Ingham T, et al: The effects of early and late paracetamol exposure on asthma and atopy: a birth cohort. Clin Exp Allergy 2011;41:399–406.
46 Rusconi F, Gagliardi L, Galassi C, Forastiere F, Brunetti L, La Grutta S, et al: Paracetamol and antibiotics in childhood and subsequent development of wheezing/asthma: association or causation? Int J Epidemiol 2011;40:662–667.

47 Lowe AJ, Carlin JB, Bennett CM, Hosking CS, Allen KJ, Robertson CF, et al: Paracetamol use in early life and asthma: prospective birth cohort study. BMJ 2010;15:341.
48 Oncel MY, Yurttutan S, Erdeve O, Uras N, Altug N, Oguz SS, et al: Oral paracetamol versus oral ibuprofen in the management of patent ductus arteriosus in preterm infants: a randomized controlled trial. J Pediatr 2014;164:510–514.
49 Dang D, Wang D, Zhang C, Zhou W, Zhou Q, Wu H: Comparison of oral paracetamol versus ibuprofen in premature infants with patent ductus arteriosus: a randomized controlled trial. PLoS One 2013; 8:e77888.
50 Hammerman C: Indomethacin and retinopathy of prematurity: The hidden paradox. J Pediatr 2008; 153:587–588.
51 NDA 21–903; Approval letter. www.accessdata.fda.gov/drugsatfda_docs/label/2006/021903lbl.pdf.

Cathy Hammerman, MD
Department of Neonatology
PO Box 3235, Shaare Zedek Med. Ctr.
Jerusalem, 91031 (Israel)
E-Mail cathyh@ekmd.huji.ac.il

Mimouni FB, van den Anker JN (eds): Neonatal Pharmacology and Nutrition Update.
Pediatr Adolesc Med. Basel, Karger, 2015, vol 18, pp 83–107 (DOI: 10.1159/000365032)

Formulation of Preterm Formula: What's in it, and Why?

Francis B. Mimouni[a, b] · Dror Mandel[b, c] · Ronit Lubetzky[b, c]

[a]Department of Neonatology, Shaare Zedek Medical Center, Jerusalem, [b]Department of Pediatrics, The Tel Aviv Medical Center, Tel Aviv, [c]Sackler School of Medicine, Tel Aviv University, Tel Aviv, Israel

Abstract

Human milk feeding of preterm infants reduces mortality and morbidity (in particular sepsis and necrotizing enterocolitis). When their own mother's milk is not available, and in the absence of donor milk, such fragile infants must be fed formula. In many instances, preterm infant formulas (PIFs) attempt to mimic the composition of human milk (the gold standard of infant feeding), but they must take into account as well the unique nutritional needs of the growing preterm infant, which are not identical to those of the healthy term infant. In this article we review the major characteristics of PIFs and try to evaluate the evidence and rationale behind their composition. A table comparing PIFs from several major manufacturers is presented for the convenience of the reader.

Introduction

In 2012, the American Academy of Pediatrics (AAP) reaffirmed its recommendation that all preterm infants should receive their mother's own milk, fresh or frozen, as their primary diet, with the provision that it should be fortified appropriately for infants born weighing less than 1.5 kg [1]. In case the mother's own milk is unavailable despite significant lactation support, the AAP advised that pasteurized donor milk should be used [1]. In the AAP position statement, the arguments in support of human milk (HM) feeding include the significant short- and long-term beneficial effects of feeding preterm infants HM, such as: lower rates of sepsis and necrotizing enterocolitis (NEC), lower mortality rates, fewer hospital readmissions for illness in the year after NICU discharge, and lower rates of long-term growth failure and neuro-developmental disabilities [1]. In spite of this statement, the use of a formula designed for premature infants might remain the only option when maternal milk is unavailable in adequate amounts and when no donor milk is available. Ob-

Table 1. Components of HM and various preterm formulas

Component (per 100 kcal)	Human milk	Term formula	SSC 24	Enfamil Premie 24	Nestle 24	Humana OH-A	Recommendations	
							minimum	maximum
Energy (Kcal)	100	100	100	100	100	100	67	94
Protein (g)	1.5	2.1	3.3	3	3.6	2.8	2.5	3.6
Carbohydrates (g)	11.9	10.9	10	11	10.1	10.3	9.6	12.5
Lactose (g)	11.9				4.6	7	4	12.5
Maltodextrin (g)					5.5	3.3		
Fat (g)	5.2	5.5	5.43	5.1	4.99	5.3	4.4	6
Linoleic acid (mg)	450	770	700	810	701	923	350	1,400
Linolenic acid (mg)		74			96	95	50	4% TF
DHA (mg)		10			18	10.6	11	0.35% TF
AA (mg)		21			18	10.6	16	0.6% TF
Calcium (mg)	45	78	180	165	145	121	110	185
Phosphorous (mg)	22.6	41	100	83	96	65	55	109
Magnesium (mg)	4.8	7.5	12	9	10.4	11	6.8	17
Iron (mg)	0.06	1.2	1.8	1.8	2.25	1.5	1.7	3
Zinc (mg)	0.38	0.7	1.5	1.5	1.5	1.1	1.1	1.8
Manganese (mcg)	1.5	19	12	6.3	16	15	6.3	25
Copper (mcg)	58	75	250	120	250	107	90	250
Iodine (mcg)	4–9	19	6	25	35	20	9	50
Selenium (mcg)		1.6	1.8	2.8	5.9	1.9	1.8	9
Sodium (mg)	22.5	27	43	58	63	48	39	105
Potassium (mg)	72.5	122	129	98	149	104	60	160
Chloride (mg)	63	65	81	90	95	68	60	161
Vitamin A	319	278 IU	1,250 IU	1,250 IU	460 mcg	116 mcg	204 mcg	740 mcg
Vitamin D (IU)	3	50 IU 1.25 mcg	150 IU	240 IU	4.67 mcg	2.5 mcg	1.8 mcg	6.75 mcg
Vitamin E (IU)	0.4	4.1 IU	4 IU	6.3 IU	4.5 mg	3.1 mg	2 mg	10 mg
Vitamin K (mcg)	0.3	9.9	12	8	8.05	8.8	4	25
Vitamin B1 (mcg)	30	120	250	200	169	146	30	275
Vitamin B2 (mcg)	50	210	620	300	247	157	80	620
Vitamin B6 (mcg)	133	60	250	150	117	117	30	273
Vitamin B12 (mcg)	0.04	0.25	0.55	0.25	0.29	0.3	0.08	0.7
Vitamin C (mg)	6	15	37	20	26	20	8.3	42
Niacin (mg)	0.21	1.04	5	4	2	2.4	0.345	5
Folic acid (mcg)	12	10	37	40	50.6	70	30	90
Pantothenic acid (mg)	0.26	0.6	1.9	1.2	1	0.88	0.3	1.9
Biotin (mcg)	0.9	37	37	4	4.9	7.2	1	37
Choline (mg)	13.4	15	10	20	25	21	7	50
Inositol (mg)		6	40	44	25	11	4	48

viously, while preterm infant formulas (PIFs) have been designed to meet the nutritional requirements of the premature infant, they cannot mimic many of the biological properties of HM. The purpose of this chapter is to review the evidence behind the composition of PIFs. We will focus on PIFs designed for the immediate postnatal (in-hospital) period and will only briefly address the issue of post-discharge formulas. A table comparing PIFs from several major manufacturers is presented for the convenience of the reader (table 1).

Fluid Intake and Energy Content

The European Society for Paediatric Gastoenterology, Hepatology and Nutrition (ESPGHAN) regards 135 ml/kg as the minimum fluid volume and 200 ml/kg as a reasonable upper limit of daily fluid intake [2]. The basis behind this recommendation is mostly an expert consensus, as 'randomised controlled trials on enteral fluid intake of "healthy" preterm infants are lacking as are studies comparing different fluid volumes providing identical nutrient intakes'. Moreover, it is believed that relatively low fluid intakes are likely to minimize the risks of bronchopulmonary dysplasia and patent ductus arteriosus. These beliefs are supported by a systematic review of 5 randomized trials evaluating varying parenteral fluid intake in premature infants, which showed that while restricted water intake significantly increased postnatal weight loss, it significantly decreased the rates of patent ductus arteriosus and NEC, bronchopulmonary dysplasia, intracranial hemorrhage and death [3]. Some infants, however, may require higher volumes to meet water (or other nutrient) requirements (particularly if insensible water losses are very high because of skin immaturity or because of the use of radiant heaters).

A few studies have been conducted that compared the growth and metabolic responses in preterm infants fed formulas with different energy contents. Generally, daily intakes ranging between 100 and 140 kcal/kg provide satisfactory growth [4, 5] while some infants, such as small for gestational age infants, may require energy intakes greater than 140 kcal/kg/day in order to grow [4]. Thus, the ESPGHAN concluded that a 'reasonable range of energy intake for healthy growing preterm infants with adequate protein intake is 110 to 135 kcal/kg/day'. In one trial, 148 extremely low-birth-weight infants with a gestational age of 23–31 weeks were evaluated for protein and energy intake in first 4 weeks of life and for the outcome at age 18 months [6]. The energy intake in the first week of life appeared to be particularly decisive for the developmental outcome, with a Mental Development Index (MDI) increased by 4.6 points for each 10 kcal/kg/day increase in energy intake ($p = 0.0134$) in first week of life. In contrast, energy intake during the following 3 weeks was not correlated with MDI [6].

Consequently, PIFs exist in various versions according to their energy content: they are mostly available at 24, 27, or even 30 kcal/oz (1 oz = 29.57 ml, i.e. approximately 30 ml). The reason why a specific energy concentration is used is essentially related to how much fluid restriction is needed for a given infant.

Protein

Protein Concentration

PIFs are designed to provide preterm infants with a higher protein intake than that provided by standard 'term' formulas. Indeed, it is widely accepted that healthy premature babies have daily protein requirements of 3.5–4.0 g/kg. A recent meta-analysis of infants born at <2,500 gm (low birth weight, or LBW) included 5 studies with 114 infants with a daily protein intake of 3–4 g/kg versus <3 g/kg [7]. Weight gain and nitrogen accretion were higher in the 3–4 g/kg group. The mean daily weight difference between the 2 groups was 2.36 g/kg (95% CI 1.31–3.4 g/kg) in favor of the higher protein intake. Two similar studies published thereafter (one in very low birth weight (VLBW) infants (birth weight (BW) <1,500 g)) [8] and one in infants with a BW <1,250 g [6] led to similar conclusions. In the previously mentioned trial of 148 extremely low-birth-weight infants (BW <1,000 g) with a gestational age of 23–31 weeks, the MDI increased 8.21 points for each 1 g/kg/day increase in protein intake in the first week of life, but the MDI was no longer influenced by protein intake during the following 3 weeks of life [9].

Protein Type

The predominant protein in HM is whey, followed by casein (80:20 ratio at the initiation of lactation decreasing to 50:50 in late lactation) [10]. PIFs are designed to be whey-dominant (60:40 ratio, usually chosen as an 'average between 80:20 and 50:50) [10]. In premature infants, whey protein is usually preferred because for the following reasons: (1) compared to casein, it is believed to promote more rapid gastric emptying, which is supported by one study [11], while in another study, we showed that gastric emptying of a casein-predominant formula was similar to that of a whey-dominant formula [12]; (2) whey is believed to be more easily digested because the whey fraction is composed of soluble proteins [10]. We must note, however, that bovine whey (with beta-lactoglobulin as its major protein) is not equivalent to human whey (with alpha-lactalbumin as its major protein), and it does not have identical amino acid composition. Subsequently, plasma concentrations of individual amino acids are different in HM-fed and PIF-fed preterm infants: infants fed HM have the lowest concentrations of methionine, phenylalanine, and tyrosine, even at daily intakes of 1.6 g/kg protein through HM compared to whey or casein-dominant formulas, which provide 2.25 or 4.50 g/kg protein [13, 14]. Additionally, PIFs are routinely supplemented with cysteine and taurine, two amino acids that are present in HM and are necessary to synthesize the antioxidant glutathione (cysteine), or for bile conjugation and brain development (taurine) [15, 16]; (3) Human whey contains important proteins that play a role in host defense, such as lactoferrin, lysozyme, and secretory IgA [17]. Once again, we note that there are only traces of these proteins in bovine milk.

In the past decade, a few PIFs have been developed based upon hydrolyzed protein. In one trial, 129 VLBW infants were randomized (without intention-to-treat analysis) to hydrolyzed protein or standard preterm formula [18]. Infants randomized to hydrolyzed protein reached full feeds in 10 days versus 12 days for those randomized to standard PIF ($p = 0.0024$) [18]. Thus, hydrolyzed protein formulas may be associated with increased feeding tolerance.

Lipids

Background

It would be extraordinarily difficult to use HM lipid composition as a model for formula lipid composition. Indeed, fats are the most variable constituents in HM, and they vary in composition over the course of a feeding (hindmilk is richer in fat than foremilk), from breast to breast, over a day's time (it is highly dependent upon maternal dietary fat intake and undergoes circadian variations), over time itself (total lipids range from approximately 2 g/dl on day 3 of lactation to approximately 5 g/dl on day 84), and among individuals [19]. In HM, fat is present as milk globules (ranging from 1 to 10 μm in diameter) whose core is composed of non-polar lipids (such as triacylglycerols) and cholesterol esters, and the outer layer (the milk-lipid-globule membrane) is made up of bipolar materials (phospholipids, proteins, cholesterol, and enzymes) that prevent the globules from coalescing and keep them in emulsion [19]. In HM, lipids provide a well-tolerated energy source (contributing about 50% of the calories); their unique composition and the presence of bile salt-stimulated lipase allow maximal intestinal absorption of fatty acids (FAs), and in addition, they provide essential fatty acids (EFAs) and polyunsaturated fatty acids (PUFAs). We will expand later on the importance of the latter two types of FA. Fatty acids are usually identified by 2 numbers, such as palmitic acid, which is identified as 16:0. The number to the left (16) represents the number of carbons, and the number to the right (0) represents the number of double bonds. Thus, in the example cited, palmitic acid is a saturated FA. In contrast, linoleic acid (18:2) has 2 double bonds and is therefore a polyunsaturated FA [19]. According to their length, FAs are classified as short chain (2–5 carbons), medium chain (6–12 carbons), and long chain (13–22 carbons) [20]. EFAs are by definition required by the human body but cannot be made in sufficient quantities from other substrates. Therefore, they must be obtained from the diet. Two major EFAs are linoleic acid (18:2) and alpha-linolenic acid (18:3), which are widely present in vegetable oils but are only present at low concentrations in cow's milk. Moreover, neonates and preterm infants have a limited ability to elongate alpha-linolenic acid into n-3 fatty acids such as eicosapentaenoic acid (EPA) and docosahexaenoic acid (DHA). These two long-chain PUFAs are present in abundance in oils obtained from fish [20]. Although fat in HM is present at a concentration very close to that in cow's milk (CM) (approximately 3.5 g/dl on average), there are striking qualitative differences: 100 g of whole cow's milk contains 2.5 g saturated fat, 1.0 g monounsaturated fat and 0.1 g polyunsaturated fat, while HM contains 1.8 g saturated fat, 1.6 g monounsaturated fat and 0.5 g polyunsaturated fat [21]. The much higher level of saturated fat in CM and the much higher level of unsaturated fat in HM make CM fat highly unsuitable for human infants. Indeed, unsaturated FAs present in HM, in particular the omega-6 fatty acid arachidonic acid (AA) and the omega-3 fatty acid DHA, play an important function in brain and retina development and function

[20]. Both AA and DHA are present in HM but not in CM. Subsequently, CM used for the production of infant formulas is defatted, and CM fat is replaced by various fat blends, mostly of vegetable origin.

Quantitative Fat Intake

The ESPGHAN recommends that the minimal daily dietary fat intake of preterm infants should be 4.8 g/kg [2]. This recommendation is based upon the fact that daily intrauterine fat deposition is 3 g/kg [22], that 10–40% of dietary fat is not absorbed, and that 15% of the fat absorbed is lost from unavoidable oxidation and conversion to deposited triglyceride in tissue [2]. The ESPGHAN states that 'at an energy intake of 110 kcal/kg, this fat intake is met by a total fat content in preterm formula of at least 4.4 g/100 kcal (or 39.5% of energy).' [2] The maximum daily dietary fat intake recommended by the ESPGHAN Committee on Nutrition is 6.0 g/100 kcal (54% of energy, E%) [22] and that recommended by the US Life Science Research Office is 5.7 g/100 kcal (51 E%) [23]. These recommendations are mostly based on expert opinion and are similar to the upper end of the range of fat concentration observed in HM. A well-documented risk of excessive fat intake is inadequate fat absorption; through soap formation, this would ultimately lead to a loss of dietary minerals [24].

Medium Chain Fatty Acids

In theory, the 'immature' preterm infant's gastrointestinal tract may have difficulties with digesting and absorbing fat from formula intake, particularly because of liver immaturity and decreased formation of bile salts, which are necessary for fat digestion [25]. In view of the fact that bile salts are not necessary for the absorption of medium chain fatty acids (MCFAs), the idea of providing them as a major source of dietary fat was particularly attractive to formula manufacturers. Thus, while MCFAs represent only 12% or less of the FAs in HM [22], most PIFs are designed to contain 40–50% of their fat as MCFAs. The evidence that has accumulated over the years did not confirm this theory. Indeed, in one study, preterm infants were randomized to formulas with 46% MCFAs or 4% MCFAs [26]. At the end of the study period, the two groups did not differ in terms of nitrogen retention, weight gain, energy expenditure, or energy storage [27]. When MCFAs are added to the diet, they might be incompletely oxidized compared to long-chain fatty acids, which could lead to milk ketosis [28]. This apparent metabolic inefficiency is seen by some as an advantage, as it may mimic the mild ketosis present in HM-fed neonates [28]. Consequently, the ESPGHAN supported the idea that if MCFAs are added to PIFs, they should not exceed 40% of the total fat content [2].

Essential Fatty Acids

As stated earlier, the two major EFAs are linoleic acid (18:2) and alpha-linolenic acid (18:3), which are widely present in vegetable oils but are present in low concentrations in cow's milk. Until now, the recommended intake of linoleic acid and alpha-linolenic acid in preterm infants has been based only on expert opinion in the absence of relevant clinical trials. While the ESPGHAN experts initially recommended linoleic acid intake in the range of 500–1,200 mg/100 kcal (4.5–10.8% of energy intake) [22], and the Life Science Research Office (LSRO) experts recommended 352–1,425 mg/100 kcal (3.2–12.8 of energy intake) [23], the ESPGHAN has updated its recommendation to an acceptable range of 385–1,540 mg/kg/day or 350–1,400 mg/100 kcal (3.2–12.6% of energy intake) [2], 500–1,200 mg/100 kcal (4.5–10.8% E%) [29], and 352–1,425 mg/100 kcal (3.2–12.8 E%) [2], equivalent to approximately 8–25% of the fatty acids in a preterm formula. There is no evidence of linoleic acid deficiency or of adverse effects from high intakes in infants fed currently available PIFs. Linoleic acid intakes of 385–1,540 mg/kg/day or 350–1,400 mg/100 kcal (3.2–12.6 E%) are considered acceptable. As far as alpha-linolenic acid (an essential precursor of EPA and DHA) is concerned, there is also a lack of scientific evidence, and the ESPGHAN experts have recommended a minimum intake of 55 mg/kg/day, or 50 mg/100 kcal (0.45% of energy intake), with a linoleic acid to alpha-linolenic acid weight ratio in the range of 5–15:1 [2]. Whether lower ranges of alpha-linolenic acid intakes might be possible when PIFs are supplemented directly with DHA is unknown.

Long-Chain Polyunsaturated Fatty Acids
Long-chain polyunsaturated fatty acids (LC-PUFAs) are important compounds for cell membrane functions and for the formation of bioactive eicosanoids. They are present in high concentrations in the grey matter of the brain and in the retina. In addition, data suggest that LC-PUFAs are beneficial for premature infants. Premature infants fed HM have much higher concentrations of AA and DHA in red blood cells than those fed formulas unsupplemented with LC-PUFAs, even if they fulfill the EFA requirements [30]. The most recent meta-analysis of trials that were conducted to study the effects of LC-PUFA supplementation in PIF was published in 2011 [30]. All 17 randomized trials of formula supplemented with LC-PUFAs that had clinical endpoints were reviewed, and 13 were classified as being of high quality. Infants enrolled in the trials were mostly relatively mature and healthy preterm infants. Visual acuity was assessed in most studies by Teller or Lea cards (8 studies), by VEP (6 studies) or by ERG (2 studies). Despite some evidence that supplementation may lead to more rapid visual information processing (more frequent shorter looks), most studies found no significant differences in visual assessment between supplemented and control infants. Meta-analysis of Bayley scales of infant development of four studies at 12 months (n = 364) and three studies at 18 months (n = 494) post-term showed no significant effects of supplementation. Meta-analysis of five studies showed increased weight and length at 2 months post-term in supplemented infants. Meta-analysis of four studies at 12 months (n = 271) and two studies at 18 months (n = 396) post-term showed no significant effect of supplementation on weight, length or head circumference. The authors of this meta-analysis concluded that the meta-analysis was limited by the fact that the assessment schedule and

methodology, the dose and source of supplementation and the fatty acid composition of the control formula varied between trials. Overall, 'no clear long-term benefits or harms were demonstrated for preterm infants receiving LCPUFA-supplemented formula'.

Nevertheless, the ESPGHAN expert committee noted that EPA competes with AA, and EPA levels are very low in HM. The committee concluded that based upon the available evidence (mostly reviewed in the above-mentioned meta-analysis that 'both AA and DHA should be included in preterm formulas, and that oils containing significant amounts of eicosapentaenoic acid should be avoided' [2]. The ESPGHAN committee suggested that 'a reasonable range for the balance between AA and DHA appears to be 1.0–2.0: 1, i.e. the range of most preterm formulas clinically tested, and similar to that found in many studies on fatty acid composition of human milk,' [2] and that EPA contents should not exceed 30% of the amount of DHA [2]. Thus, they recommend a dietary intake of 12–30 mg/kg/day or 11–27 mg/100 kcal for DHA (22: 6n-3) and of 18–42 mg/kg/day or 16–39 mg/100 kcal for AA (20:4n-6) [2].

Carbohydrates

Background

Carbohydrates contribute about 40% of the caloric content of HM. Carbohydrates in HM are mostly lactose and oligosaccharides. In term infants, more than 90% of the lactose from HM is absorbed, leaving only a small amount to reach the colon, where it promotes the growth of intestinal flora and softer stool consistency [31]. Lactose is also known to promote mineral absorption [32]. However, because of reduced lactase production compared to that in term infants [33], preterm infants do not have similarly efficient lactose absorption. In preterm infants, approximately 80% of lactose is absorbed [34]. Unabsorbed lactose reaches the colon, where it can be partly 'salvaged' by fermentation and absorbed as short-chain fatty acids, lactate or other organic acids [35]. The salvage might not be complete, as a randomized controlled trial of lactase in preterm infants at 26–34 weeks of gestation showed increased weight gain in the lactase-supplemented group [36].

Quantitative Requirements

Minimum and maximum daily carbohydrate requirements have been recommended by the ESPGHAN (expert consensus) [2]. These limits have been calculated on the basis that carbohydrates must provide the total energy requirements minus the calories of the protein and fat requirements. Assuming that protein provides 12% of the calories from formula and that fat provides 40% of the calories, the ESPGHAN expert committee suggested that the remaining 48% should be provided by carbohydrates, i.e. at a minimum concentration of 10.5 g/100 kcal and at a maximum concentration of 12.0 g/100 kcal [2].

Types of Carbohydrates
Carbohydrates in PIF are usually composed of equal parts lactose and a polymer of glucose. An obvious advantage of this composition, in spite of its departure from the HM model, is the fact that it reduces the osmotic load of the formula. Another theoretical advantage is that it does not overwhelm the lactase-producing capabilities of the immature gut. Moreover, it appears that such a mixture of carbohydrates does not impair mineral absorption [29]. Reducing the amount of lactose in PIF might be beneficial in terms of feeding tolerance [37]. One study of 306 infants born at less than 36 weeks gestation and at a birth weight of less than 1,800 g compared those randomized to a low-lactose formula (<5% lactose) vs. a lactose-containing formula [37]. The low-lactose formula was associated with improved feeding tolerance (decreased mean time to achieve full feeds), greater enteral caloric intake, and greater daily weight gain without affecting the rates of NEC [37]. Thus, currently available PIFs contain 4–7 g lactose/100 kcal (while HM contains approximately 10 g lactose/100 kcal) [2].

Minerals

Calcium, Phosphorus and Magnesium Requirements
It cannot be assumed that HM, which is designed to fit the extrauterine requirements of the term infant, can be used as an ideal model for the preterm infant. Intrauterine and extrauterine growth and nutrient accretion rates are not identical. Mineral requirements of the preterm infant are subsequently estimated on the basis of two major assumptions: the first one is related to the estimated intrauterine mineral accretion rate, and the other one relates to the degree of intestinal mineral absorption by the preterm infant. All expert opinions on this topic are based on these 2 assumptions, whether they are the 1987 ESPGHAN recommendations [38], commented upon and revised in 2009 [2], the LSRO recommendations [23], the Atkinson and Tsang recommendations [39], or the Rigo et al. recommendations [40]. Mineral accretion estimates during pregnancy are essentially all based upon the cornerstone studies of Widdowson [41], who analyzed the chemical composition of fetuses at various gestational ages. According to Widdowson, during the last 3 months of gestation, the fetal accretion of calcium (Ca) and phosphorus (P) is about 20 and 10 g, respectively, which represents accretion rates of approximately 100–120 mg/kg/day for Ca, 50–65 mg/kg/day for P, while the accretion rate is 3–5 mg/day for magnesium (Mg) [41].

The assumptions used for intestinal absorption estimates in the above-mentioned recommendations are based upon either older balance studies or upon studies using stable isotopes of Ca and Mg [42]. Although these studies have greatly improved our knowledge of mineral metabolism and balance, they have shown that there is significant variability of mineral absorption among preterm infants. The coefficient of absorption of Ca ranges grossly between 50 and 70% and that of P between 60 and 90% [43]. These variations alone explain most of the differences among the various expert recommendations. The lowest estimate for Ca requirements in mg/kg/day is that of the ESPGHAN [38], and the highest is that of the LSRO [23]. Similarly, the lowest estimate for P requirements is that of the ESPGHAN [38], and the highest is that of Atkinson [39]. Most of the recent data using stable isotopes of Ca [43] are consistent with relatively lower coefficients of absorption of Ca than those shown by the older data; thus, they favor the higher estimates as proposed by Atkinson. Thus, daily requirements for Ca should be 120–200 mg/kg. The ESPGHAN [2] used an estimate of a 90% coefficient of absorption for P, an optimistic estimate when considering, for instance, the data by Lapillonne, who found coefficients of absorption of 76% in fortified HM-fed preterm infants and 65.3% in those fed a preterm formula [44]. Thus, daily requirements for P should be higher than those that are currently recommended by the ESPGHAN and similar to the Atkinson and Tsang proposals (60–140 mg/kg).

In HM, the Ca:P ratio is 2:1 in mass, close to the actual composition of skeletal minerals (2.2:1) [2]. It is therefore recommended that the Ca:P ratio (by weight) be maintained approximately at the level present in HM, i.e. approximately 2:1.

Preterm infants fed HM are provided with a Mg intake of 5.5–7.5 mg/kg/day. The ESPGHAN assumed an absorption coefficient of 40%, and calculated a net accretion of 2.2–3 mg/kg/day, i.e. less than the 3–5 mg/kg/day of intrauterine accretion (for a 1-kg baby) [2]. It recommended that infants fed formula be provided with Mg intakes of 8–12 mg/kg/day because they had a retention rate within the range of intrauterine accretion [45]. Lapillonne et al. found a 37.5% coefficient of absorption for Mg in their balance studies both in fortified HM fed preterm infants and in those fed a preterm formula [44]. In contrast, Koo and Tsang assumed that the coefficient of absorption of Mg was 50% and thus estimated the requirements to be 8 mg/kg/day (0.33 mmol) [46]. In view of a more realistic coefficient of absorption of approximately 40% [44, 47], the daily requirements for Mg should be 8–12 mg/kg, as suggested by ESPGHAN [2].

In general, PIFs given at a daily volume of 150 ml/kg/day provide daily intakes of approximately 200 mg/kg Ca or more and 100 mg/kg P, which meet the above-mentioned estimates of intrauterine accretion. It is obvious that formulas designed for term infants do not and cannot meet the mineral requirements of premature infants.

Sodium

Sodium (Na) is fundamental for maintenance of extracellular fluid volume and blood pressure regulation. An adequate intake should allow for adequate growth and maintenance of serum Na within an adequate range. The Na concentration of HM is very low, and at times, premature infants fed HM exclusively become hyponatremic [48]. The ESPGHAN recommends that the minimum and maximum Na intake should be, respectively, 63 mg/100 kcal (approximately 2.7 mmol/100 kcal) and 85 mg/100 kcal (approximately 4.6 mmol/100 kcal).

Potassium

Potassium (K) is the most abundant intracellular cation. It plays a major role in the maintenance of transmembrane electrical potential and intestinal ionic strength. It is therefore critical for cardiac contractility, blood pressure regulation and nerve function. The ESPGHAN recommends that the minimum daily K intake should be 60 mg/100 kcal, and the maximum daily K intake should be 120 mg/100 kcal (≈1.5–3.1 mmol/100 kcal) [2]. This amount is amply provided by both HM and PIF.

Iron

Iron (Fe) is not only essential to hemoglobin and myoglobin formation, it also appears to be essential to brain development. Iron deficiency anemia has been associated with poor neurodevelopmental outcomes [49]. Thus it would appear that Fe deficiency is critical to avoid in preterm infants. However, Fe is a potent pro-oxidant and, when given in excess, it has the potential for harm [50]. At birth, total body Fe approximates 75 mg/kg [41], which is equivalent to a daily accretion rate of 1–1.5 mg/kg/day. In VLBW infants, another cause of Fe deficiency is Fe loss due to phlebotomy, which may approximate 6 mg/kg per week [51], while each blood transfusion is estimated to provide an Fe load of approximately 8 mg/kg [2]. Iron absorption from preterm formula may be as low as 11% [52], much less than the 50% figure reported for HM [53, 54]. The Fe concentration in HM is relatively low and continues to decline over lactation (from about 0.6 mg/l at 2 weeks to 0.3 mg/l after 5 months) [55].

In view of the fact that an Fe intake of <2 mg/kg/day is likely to result in Fe deficiency in preterm infants and that high enteral Fe intake has been associated with possible adverse effects, the ESPGHAN recommends an intake of 2–3 mg/kg/day, corresponding to 1.8–2.7 mg/100 kcal [2]. In contrast, the AAP recommends a higher upper limit, with an intake of 2–4 mg/kg/day [56]. Nevertheless, in order to provide such intakes, all PIFs should be unquestionably Fe fortified.

Zinc

Zinc (Zn) is the cofactor of many enzymes and is important for cell growth and differentiation. During the last trimester of pregnancy, the fetal Zn accretion rate approximates 0.85 mg/day, or 35 μg/g weight gain [57]. Typically, the main consequences of Zn deficiency are growth failure, susceptibility to infections, a peculiar skin rash, and delayed neurodevelopment [58]. Preterm infants absorb 30–40% of ingested Zn, with better absorption of Zn from HM than from formula [59, 60]. The Zn content in HM declines over time, from 5.4 mg/l of colostrum, to 1.1 mg/l after 3 months [61].

Using the factorial method, dietary Zn requirements for preterm infants have been calculated as 1–2 mg/kg/day [23]. The ESPGHAN suggests a Zn intake of 1.1–2.0 mg/kg/day or 1.0–1.8 mg/100 kcal [2]. In most PIFs, Zn concentration approximates 1.25 mg/dl (nearly 10 times more than mature HM), which should be sufficient to match a retention equivalent to intrauterine accretion rates [62].

Copper

Copper (Cu) is also a cofactor for various enzymatic systems, in particular the antioxidant copper/zinc superoxide dismutase (CuZn-SOD) [63]. The daily Cu fetal accretion rate is approximately 50 μg/kg [57]. Similarly to that of Zn, the Cu content in HM decreases over lactation from 600 μg/l during the first week to 220 μg/l by 5 months [64]. Approximately 60% of the Cu in HM is absorbed compared to 16% of the Cu in cow's milk [59]. The minimum daily dietary Cu requirement for preterm infants has been estimated to be 100 μg/kg [23]. The ESPGHAN recommends a daily Cu intake of 100–132 μg/kg or 90–120 μg/100 kcal. Most PIFs provide a Cu intake of 200–300 μg/kg/day, which is higher than the fetal accretion rates [65].

Selenium

Selenium (Se) is an essential trace element that is part of a number of selenoproteins including glutathione peroxidase, an enzyme important in protecting against oxidative damage [66]. Blood Se is lower in preterm than in term infants [66]. Very preterm infants with low Se concentrations have an increased risk of bronchopulmonary dysplasia and retinopathy of prematurity [66]. One Cochrane review of the studies using Se supplementation to prevent short-term morbidity in preterm neonates found 3 eligible trials. Meta-analysis of the pooled data showed a significant reduction in the proportion of infants having one or more episodes of sepsis associated with Se supplementation. Selenium supplementation of at least 5 μg/kg/day is necessary to maintain blood Se concentration close to the range of that of umbilical concentrations [67]. The ESPGHAN recommends that the Se intake for preterm infants should be 5–10 μg/kg/day or 4.5–9 μg/100 kcal [2].

Vitamins

Thiamin (Vitamin B1)
Thiamin is a fundamental coenzyme for energy metabolism. Studies in preterm infants show that thiamin content in HM is not sufficient to maintain an adequate thiamine status [68, 69]. The younger the gestational age, the lower the birth weight and the lower the thiamin status [70]. The ESPGHAN recommends a daily thiamin intake

of 140–300 μg/kg/day or 125–275 μg/100 kcal [2]. With current feeding practices of preterm infants, which include the use of PIF, thiamin deficiency is usually prevented [70].

Riboflavin (Vitamin B2)
Riboflavin is the central component of the cofactors FAD and FMN and is required by all flavoproteins. It plays a key role in energy metabolism and in the metabolism of fats, ketone bodies, carbohydrates, and proteins. In humans, signs and symptoms of riboflavin deficiency include gastrointestinal mucosal damage. However, when given in excess, flavins are thought to contribute to oxidative stress through their ability to produce superoxide [71]. Based on biochemical indices, a minimal intake of 200 μg/kg/day is needed to ensure normal riboflavin status in preterm infants [68, 69]. Adequate riboflavin status of preterm infants is supported by an average intake of 300 μg/kg/day [68, 69]. Higher intakes (i.e. 670 μg/100 kcal [68] may result in low erythrocyte glutathione reductase activity [72]. Thus, the ESPGHAN recommends that the riboflavin content of PIF should not exceed two times the minimum level and should range between 200 and 400 μg/kg/day or between 180 and 365 μg/100 kcal [2].

Niacin (Vitamin B3)
Niacin is a water-soluble organic compound with the formula $C_6H_5NO_2$. Niacin can be converted to NAD and NADP. These are coenzymes of many hydrogenases that play an important role in hydrogen transfer. Thus, niacin is involved in the metabolism of fat, carbohydrates, and proteins, and it is involved in DNA repair. In humans, niacin deficiency causes pellagra, with diarrhea, dermatitis, and dementia. The niacin requirements of preterm infants have not been systematically studied. The LSRO and the ESPGHAN recommended dietary intake of niacin ranges from 380 to 5,500 μg/kg/day or from 345 to 5,000 μg/100 kcal [2].

Pantothenic Acid (Vitamin B5)
Pantothenic acid, a water-soluble vitamin, is required to synthesize coenzyme-A and is critical to the synthesis and metabolism of proteins, carbohydrates, and fats. Only the D isomer has biological activity. In humans, deficiency is rare and is characterized by irritability and fatigue, various neurological symptoms, increased insulin sensitivity, and hypoglycemia, as well as by gastrointestinal symptoms. Preterm infants fed HM do not present with signs of pantothenic deficiency; thus, the LSRO and the ESPGHAN recommend a pantothenic acid intake of 0.33–2.1 mg/kg/day or 0.3–1.9 mg/100 kcal [2].

Pyridoxine (Vitamin B6)
As a cofactor of aromatic amino acid decarboxylase, pyridoxine is required for the synthesis of neurotransmitters such as serotonin, dopamine, norepinephrine, and epinephrine. It is important in the metabolism of Na and K and is involved in red

blood cell production. In humans, pyridoxine deficiency may lead to anemia, to CNS symptoms such as seizures, and to mucocutaneous damage. HM contains 70–310 μg pyridoxine/l (10.4–46.3 μg/100 kcal) [73]. Because a daily intake of pyridoxine of 300 μg/kg/day was not associated with any untoward side effects [74], and an intake of 4.3 μg/g protein resulted in deficiency symptoms [75], the ESPGHAN recommended an intake of 45–300 μg/kg/day or 41–330 μg/100 kcal.

Cobalamin (Vitamin B12)

Cobalamin is a water-soluble compound that plays a critical role in hematopoiesis and in brain function. Because it affects DNA synthesis and regulation, it affects essentially every single cell in the human body. Its name derives from its content of cobalt, a relatively rare element. Cobalamin deficiency can cause irreversible damage to the nervous system and is the cause of severe anemia. An excess of vitamin B12 is usually very well tolerated. Hepatic storage of vitamin B12 in preterm infants is less than that reported in term infants [76]; despite this reduced storage, there are no reports of vitamin B12 deficiency in preterm infants fed HM. Thus, the ESPGHAN took into consideration the average HM contents [77] and recommends a vitamin B12 intake of 0.1–0.77 μg/kg/day or 0.08–0.7 μg/100 kcal. Higher values (3 μg/kg/day) might be recommended in infants treated with erythropoietin and Fe supplements [78].

Folic Acid (Folate, or Vitamin B9)

Folic acid is a water-soluble compound that becomes biologically active after conversion to folate (also known as vitamin M, vitamin B9, vitamin Bc (or folacin), pteroyl-L-glutamic acid, pteroyl-L-glutamate, and pteroylmonoglutamic acid). Folate is composed of an aromatic pteridine ring linked to para-aminobenzoic acid and one or more glutamate residues. Folic acid is itself not biologically active, but it becomes active after its conversion in the liver to dihydrofolic acid and then to tetrahydrofolate and other derivatives. Folate is needed for DNA synthesis, repair, and methylation, hence its importance in cell division and growth. In embryos, folic acid deficiency leads to higher rates of neural tube defects, and in children and adults, it leads to diarrhea, macrocytic anemia, weakness and peripheral neuropathy. A minimum intake of 30–40 μg/kg/day has been required to prevent deficiency in preterm infants [68, 69]. The ESPGHAN recommended a folic acid intake of 35–100 μg/kg/day or 32–90 μg folic acid/100 kcal [2]. Higher values (100 μg/kg/day) might be required in infants treated with erythropoietin and Fe supplements [78].

L-Ascorbic Acid (Vitamin C)

Ascorbic acid is a water-soluble compound with potent antioxidant properties. It is capable of terminating chain radical reactions generated by oxygen radicals by electron transfer. Human vitamin C deficiency (scurvy) is characterized by multiple signs and symptoms related to deficient collagen formation, particularly skin spots, tooth loss from spongy gums, mucous membrane bleeding, and decreased resistance to infections. In term infants, the minimum recommended formula concentration of vitamin C is 10 mg/100 kcal [79]. In preterm infants given a daily average of 28 mg/kg, there were adequate plasma vitamin C concentrations [69]. A randomized controlled trial comparing a high dose (40–46 mg/kg/day) versus a 'standard' dose of vitamin C (20–26 mg/kg/day) showed a reduction in rate of bronchopulmonary dysplasia at 36 weeks postmenstrual age in the high-intake group [80]. Thus, the ESPGHAN recommends a daily vitamin C intake of 11–46 mg/kg/day or 10–42 mg/100 kcal [2].

Biotin

Biotin (or vitamin H, coenzyme R, or vitamin B7) is a water-soluble compound that acts as a coenzyme for carboxylase enzymes. It is important in the synthesis of fatty acids, isoleucine, and valine and in gluconeogenesis. Biotin deficiency is rare because biotin is produced by intestinal bacteria. In humans, biotin deficiency may cause alopecia, conjunctivitis, and a scaly, red rash in periorbital, perioral, and genital areas, as well as neurological symptoms. There are no data that allow the clear definition of biotin requirements for preterm infants. Currently available PIFs contain very large amounts of biotin when compared to HM, which contains 0.75–1.3 μg/100 kcal [77]. No adverse effects have been reported that may be related to biotin excess in these infants. Thus, the ESPGHAN recommends a biotin intake for preterm infants of 1.7–16.5 μg/kg/day or 1.5–15 μg/100 kcal [2].

Vitamin A

Like all other fat-soluble vitamins, vitamin A is absorbed with dietary fat and is primarily stored in liver and fat tissue. Because of their limited amount of fat tissue and their rapid growth, preterm infants are prone to deficiency of fat-soluble vitamins (A, D, E, and K). Vitamin A includes several molecules, among which beta-carotene is the most important. It is critical for adequate growth and development, for adequate immune function, and for night vision. Small preterm infants have lower blood values at birth than term infants, and further vitamin A absorption might be impaired by decreased bile formation. HM contains approximately 120–180 μg RE (retinol-equivalent)/l that might not be sufficient to support the needs of a preterm infant. Because of the antioxidant properties of vitamin A, its deficiency might be a risk factor for bronchopulmonary dysplasia [81]. The ESPGHAN considered the upper and lower limits of vitamin intake A to be 400–1,000 μg RE/kg/day (1,330–3,330 IU vit A/kg/day) or 360–740 μg/100 kcal (1,210–2,466 IU vit A/100 kcal), provided as preformed vitamin A [2].

Vitamin E

Vitamin E is a group of fat-soluble compounds (tocopherols and tocotrienols). The most biologically active form of vitamin E is alpha-tocopherol. It acts as an antioxidant and is found in all tissues. At birth, preterm infants, who are nearly devoid of fat, have lower vitamin E reserves because 90% of the tocopherol is located in fat tissue. In preterm infants, vitamin E deficiency is known to cause hemolytic anemia aggravated by Fe (an oxidant) supply [82]. The ESPGHAN recommends a daily supply of vitamin E of in preterm infants of 2.2 to 11 mg alpha-TE (alpha-tocopherol equivalent)/kg/day [2], or 2–10 mg alpha-TE/100 kcal [2].

Vitamin K

Vitamin K is a group of fat-soluble 2-methyl-1,4-naphthoquinone (3-) derivatives critical for posttranslational activation of proteins involved in blood coagulation, bone formation and other tissue functions. Vitamin K induces the carboxylation of glutamate residues of these proteins to form gamma-carboxyglutamate (Gla) residues, usually involved in binding Ca, which confers on them their biological activity. In humans, deficiency is mostly evidenced by a bleeding tendency. Newborn infants, particularly those who are breastfed, are at an increased risk of deficiency and the so-called 'hemorrhagic disease of the newborn', which has been practically eradicated since the introduction of routine administration of high doses of vitamin K without toxicity [83, 84]. The ESPGHAN recommends, assuming that prophylactic vitamin K1 is administered within hours of birth, that PIF should provide 4.4–28 μg/kg/day or 4–25 μg/100 kcal [2].

Vitamin D

Vitamin D is a group of fat-soluble secosteroids that mediate the intestinal absorption of Ca and P. Vitamin D is not, strictly speaking, a vitamin because human skin exposed to ultraviolet B from the sun can synthesize it. Moreover, it is a pro-hormone because it needs to be hydroxylated in the liver on carbon 25 and in the kidney on carbon 1 in order to achieve its full biological activity. The end-product, calcitriol (or 1,25 OH2 vitamin D) has many other functions unrelated to bone; it plays an important role in cell proliferation, differentiation, and apoptosis and is important for neuromuscular function, inflammation, and as an immunomodulator. Vitamin D deficiency may present as rickets (in growing infants) or as osteomalacia (in adults). The issue of the vitamin D requirements of preterm infants is complex. Indeed, the requirements might be affected by mineral availability. Whether all the elements of adequate vitamin D metabolism (including production, absorption, action and degradation) are mature and functional in preterm infants is controversial. At birth, vitamin D stores (as estimated from serum 25 OH vitamin D concentrations) correlate with maternal serum concentrations and are mostly influenced by maternal race, sun exposure and dietary intake rather than GA at birth [85]. Specific populations, such as sub-continental Indian [86], Middle-Eastern Arab [87] and to a certain extent, African-American preterm infants [88], are at a greater risk of vitamin D deficiency at birth. Vitamin D skin production has never been studied in preterm infants. Preterm infants are not likely to be exposed to UVB during their NICU stay and are not likely to not be routinely exposed to

UVB after discharge without using sunblock [89]. Thus, the vitamin D status of preterm infants is essentially dependent on vitamin D dietary intake. Studies on preterm infants given doses as low as 108 IU/day [90] and as high as 1,000 IU/day [91] show that preterm infants have increases in serum 25 OH D concentrations similar to those of term infants, which supports the concept of similar vitamin D absorption (and 25 hydroxylation). With daily intakes of 400 IU, 87% of preterm infants achieve 25 OH D concentrations above 50 nmol/l (20 ng/ml), a level that meets requirements in terms of skeletal health, and 8% achieve concentrations above 125 nmol/l, a level associated with potential risk of harm [92]. In one study from Japan, where PIFs have very high vitamin D contents, as high as 2,700 IU/l, 75% of serum samples obtained from preterm infants had 25 OH D values above 100 nmol/l [93]. Importantly, in these infants, urinary Ca/creatinine ratios were not reliable indicators of excessive vitamin D intake [93]. Many studies have shown adequate 25 OH D increases after administration of vitamin D in preterm infants [90, 91, 94–96], which supports the concept that both the absorption and the 25 hydroxylation of vitamin D are adequate. Most studies have reported higher values of 1,25 OH2 D in preterm infants than in term infants [97]. Those infants with rickets of prematurity and/or fractures actually have the highest values [97, 98]. Thus, it appears that the regulation of renal 1-hydroxylation is effective and is in place in small preterm infants. Ravid et al. [99] suggested that the in vitro 1,25 OH2 D effect on lymphocytes is blunted compared to that in adults. However, in their study, there were no differences between lymphocytes obtained from term infants and those obtained from preterm infants. Thus, there is no strong evidence that the metabolism of vitamin D in preterm infants is different from that in term infants. Moreover, the mean serum 25 OH D concentrations in small preterm infants with rickets or fractures are not different from those of preterm infants without rickets or fractures. In 1989, Evans and collaborators [100] randomized 81 small preterm infants to 400 IU versus 200 IU of vitamin D daily, and 2 months later, they did not find any differences in bone outcome. Koo et al. randomized VLBW infants fed high Ca and high P preterm formula to a daily vitamin D intake of 200, 400 or 800 IU [101]. They found no biochemical or radiological differences between the groups. Backstrom et al. randomized preterm infants to 500 versus 1,000 IU daily and reported no difference in bone mass between the groups at either 3 months [102] or at age 11 years [103]. In a recent study, 48 preterm infants were randomized to 3 groups with different vitamin D intakes (200, 400, or 800 IU daily) [104]. Serum Ca and P were not different among groups after 2 weeks of treatment, and serum osteocalcin (an index of bone formation and turnover) increased similarly in all 3 groups. The highest intake group had a significant increase in urine deoxypyridinoline, an index of bone resorption [104]. This study was small and did not attempt to directly study bone density. Finally, a comparative study of 32 preterm infants with enamel defects and 64 controls failed to demonstrate that a daily vitamin D dose of 500 IU or 100 IU could reduce the prevalence of such defects

[105]. Thus, it appears that recommendations for vitamin D intake of preterm infants should not differ from that of term infants and should be consistent with the current AAP recommendations to provide infants with a daily dose of 400 IU during the first year of life [106]. This dose is probably sufficient to maintain adequate (>50 nmol/l) serum concentrations of 25 OH D in most preterm infants and to prevent vitamin D deficiency rickets without exposing them to significant risks of vitamin D intoxication. Whether or not it is also sufficient to provide infants with extra-skeletal benefits of vitamin D is not known at this moment [85].

Other Compounds

Nucleotides

A nucleotide is an organic molecule composed of a nucleotide base, a five-carbon sugar (ribose or deoxyribose), and at least one phosphate group. Nucleotides (NT) make up the basic units of DNA and RNA molecules. NT are essential compounds of the energy transfer systems (i.e. in adenosine and guanosine triphosphate) [107]. Dietary NT have been reported to enhance small intestinal development and to modify intestinal microflora, blood lipids and immune responses [2].

HM has a wide range of nucleotide contents that are generally higher than those of bovine milk, which is the source of most infant formulas. As the composition of HM is considered the gold standard, NT have been added to some term formulas in the US since the mid-1980s and to preterm formula since 2002. Recently, the proportion of formulas that are supplemented with NT is increasing without any reported negative side effects [2, 108].

The primary justification for these additions was evidence in animals and in humans that dietary NT enhance the development of the gastrointestinal and immune systems [109, 110].

Although thirteen NT have been described in HM, only five have been added to infant formulas. The hypothesis that NT are semi-essential nutrients needs to be further evaluated, particularly in the presence of prematurity. The available preclinical and clinical studies do not provide convincing justification for the addition of nucleotides to PIF. In case nucleotides are added, the total amount should not exceed 5 mg/100 kcal, as is recommended for term formulas [2].

Choline

Choline is a water-soluble essential nutrient, appears in the head groups of phosphatidylcholine and sphingomyelin (essential constituents of membranes), and is the precursor molecule for the neurotransmitter acetylcholine, which influences the function of the brain, heart, muscle, adrenal gland, and gastrointestinal tract, as well as many other organs [111]. Large amounts of choline are required in neonates for rapid organ growth and membrane biosynthesis. HM contains choline in the form of choline, phosphocholine, glycerophosphocholine, sphingomyelin, and phosphatidylcholine [112].

Neonates consume only a single food – milk – that contains high and changing concentrations of choline. Cow's milk-based infant formulas contain 40–150 μmol/dl choline, depending on the protein source, and soy formulas contain about 120 μmol/dl [2].

There are no data to recommend an optimal intake of choline in premature infants.

Based on the limited available information on the optimal intake of choline by premature infants, it is recommended that preterm infants receive a choline supply of 8–55 mg/kg/day or 7–50 mg/100 kcal [2].

Inositol

Inositol is a chemical compound with formula $C_6H_{12}O_6$, a sixfold alcohol of cyclohexane. It exists in nine possible stereoisomers; the most prominent form is *myo*-inositol. *myo*-Inositol plays an important role as the structural basis for a number of secondary messengers in eukaryotic cells. Inositol serves as an important component of the structural lipids phosphatidylinositol and its various phosphates, the phosphatidylinositol phosphate lipids [113].

The concentration of *myo*-inositol in HM is comparable with those of some macroelements such as Na and chloride and higher than those of vitamins and trace elements [114].

It may be that the role of *myo*-inositol in neonatal nutrition has been underestimated. Preliminary data showed that the serum concentration of *myo*-inositol in newborns remains high through the early months of life, decreasing to adult concentrations by age 3–6 months [115].

Alterations in serum concentrations of *myo*-inositol have been linked to the pathogenesis of diabetic neuropathy and to the regulation of surfactant synthesis in newborn infants with respiratory distress syndrome [116, 117].

The essentiality of dietary *myo*-inositol for term and preterm infants remains an open question, although it is an essential nutrient for at least two other species of mammals.

There are relatively high levels of inositol in cord blood and in the blood of preterm infants, suggesting that it plays an important role in prenatal and neonatal development [114, 115].

A potential benefit of inositol supplementation has been reported for surfactant production and lung development as well as for protection against the development of retinopathy of prematurity [118, 119].

The concentration of *myo*-inositol in HM ranges from about 13–48 mg/100 kcal.

Until more data are available, a minimum content of 4 mg/100 kcal and an upper limit that should not exceed that found in mature HM (48 mg/100 kcal) are recommended [2].

The Future of Preterm Infant Formula

Pre- and Probiotics

Preterm infants have immature physiological systems and an underdeveloped gastrointestinal barrier function, as reflected by increased intestinal permeability. Digestive and absorptive capabilities are also decreased due to low concentrations of lactase, pancreatic lipase and bile salts [120]. Preterm infants in neonatal intensive care units develop a different intestinal microbiota compared to healthy breastfed infants due to decreased exposure to the maternal microbiota, increased exposure to organisms that colonize intensive care units, multiple courses of antibiotics, and delays in feeding [121]. This different flora makes the preterm infant more susceptible to antibiotic-resistant infections, systemic inflammatory response syndrome, and NEC [2].

Probiotics

Probiotics are defined as 'live microorganisms' that, when administered in adequate amounts, confer a health benefit to the host. Health benefits conferred by probiotic bacteria are strain specific, and there are a number of ways in which probiotics improve health [122].

Some studies and meta-analyses showed a lower risk of NEC for preterm infants receiving probiotics supplementation compared to controls. The risk for sepsis or all-cause mortality and the time to reach full feeds were also evaluated under probiotic treatment and showed conflicting results [123].

Currently, the most effective probiotic or combination, dosage and timing of probiotic supplementation is unknown, while safety issues regarding the introduction of potentially infectious agents to immature infants are not defined as risk free [2]. At this point, there is no recommendation for the use of probiotic supplements in preterm infants [2].

Prebiotics

Prebiotics are non-digestible oligosaccharides that benefit the host by selectively stimulating the growth and/or activity of beneficial bacteria in the colon and improving the host's health [124]. HM contains more than 130 different oligosaccharides implicated in maintaining normal gut flora and in inhibiting the growth of pathogenic bacteria [2]. It has been hypothesized that oligosaccharides may accelerate feeding advancement, reduce the incidence of gastrointestinal complications such as NEC, improve immunological functions, reduce the incidence of hospital-acquired infections, and improve long-term outcomes, but there are no data available from preterm studies to support these assumptions [2]. Further trials relating to the efficacy and safety of prebiotics in preterm infants should be conducted. The presently available data do not permit recommending the routine use of prebiotics as food supplements in preterm infants [2].

References

1 American Academy of Pediatrics, Section on Breastfeeding: Breast feeding and the use of human milk. Pediatrics 2012;129:e827–e841.

2 Agostoni C, Buonocore G, Carnielli VP, De Curtis M, Darmaun D, Decsi T, Domellöf M, Embleton ND, Fusch C, Genzel-Boroviczeny O, Goulet O, Kalhan SC, Kolacek S, Koletzko B, Lapillonne A, Mihatsch W, Moreno L, Neu J, Poindexter B, Puntis J, Putet G, Rigo J, Riskin A, Salle B, Sauer P, Shamir R, Szajewska H, Thureen P, Turck D, van Goudoever JB, Ziegler EE; ESPGHAN Committee on Nutrition: Enteral nutrient supply for preterm infants: commentary from the European Society of Paediatric Gastroenterology, Hepatology and Nutrition Committee on Nutrition. J Pediatr Gastroenterol Nutr 2010;50:85–91.

3 Bell EF, Acarregui MJ: Restricted versus liberal water intake for preventing morbidity and mortality in preterm infants. Cochrane Database Syst Rev 2008; CD000503.

4 Van Goudoever JB, Sulkers EJ, Lafeber HN, Sauer PJ: Short-term growth and substrate use in very-low-birth-weight infants fed formulas with different energy contents. Am J Clin Nutr 2000;71:816–821.

5 Kashyap S, Forsyth M, Zucker C, Ramakrishnan R, Dell RB, Heird WC: Effects of varying protein and energy intakes on growth and metabolic response in low birth weight infants. J Pediatr 1986;108:955–963.

6 Stephens BE, Walden RV, Gargus RA, Tucker R, McKinley L, Mance M, Nye J, Vohr BR: First-week protein and energy intakes are associated with 18-month developmental outcomes in extremely low birth weight infants. Pediatrics 2009;123:1337–1343.

7 Premji SS, Fenton TR, Sauve RS: Higher versus lower protein intake in formula-fed low birth weight infants. Cochrane Database Syst Rev 2006; CD003959.

8 Cooke R, Embleton N, Rigo J, Carrie A, Haschke F, Ziegler E: High protein pre-term infant formula: effect on nutrient balance, metabolic status and growth. Pediatr Res 2006;59:265–270.

9 Brumberg HL, Kowalski L, Troxell-Dorgan A, Gettner P, Konstantino M, Poulsen JF, Ehrenkranz RA: Randomized trial of enteral protein and energy supplementation in infants less than or equal to 1,250 g at birth. J Perinatol 2010;30:517–521.

10 Lönnerdal B: Nutritional and physiologic significance of human milk proteins. Am J Clin Nutr 2003; 77:1537S–1543S.

11 Billeaud C, Guillet J, Sandler B: Gastric emptying in infants with or without gastro-oesophageal reflux according to the type of milk. Eur J Clin Nutr 1990;44: 577–583.

12 Thorkelsson T, Mimouni F, Namgung R, Fernández-Ulloa M, Krug-Wispé S, Tsang RC: Similar gastric emptying rates for casein- and whey-predominant formulas in preterm infants. Pediatr Res 1994; 36:329–333.

13 Gaull GE, Rassin DK, Räihä NC, Heinonen K: Milk protein quantity and quality in low-birth-weight infants. III. Effects on sulfur amino acids in plasma and urine. J Pediatr 1977;90:348–355.

14 Rassin DK, Gaull GE, Räihä NC, Heinonen K: Milk protein quantity and quality in low-birth-weight infants. IV. Effects on tyrosine and phenylalanine in plasma and urine. J Pediatr 1977;90:356–360.

15 Viña J, Vento M, García-Sala F, Puertes IR, Gascó E, Sastre J, Asensi M, Pallardó FV: L-cysteine and glutathione metabolism are impaired in premature infants due to cystathionase deficiency. Am J Clin Nutr 1995;61:1067–1069.

16 Chesney RW, Helms RA, Christensen M, Budreau AM, Han X, Sturman JA: The role of taurine in infant nutrition. Adv Exp Med Biol 1998;442:463–476.

17 Goldblum RM, Schanler RJ, Garza C, Goldman AS: Human milk feeding enhances the urinary excretion of immunologic factors in low birth weight infants. Pediatr Res 1989;25:184–188.

18 Mihatsch WA, Franz AR, Högel J, Pohlandt F: Hydrolyzed protein accelerates feeding advancement in very low birth weight infants. Pediatrics 2002;110: 1199–1203.

19 Lawrence RA, Lawrence RM: Biochemistry of human milk; in Lawrence RA, Lawrence RM (eds): Breastfeeding, a Guide for the Medical Profession, ed 5. St Louis, Mosby, 1999, pp 95–158.

20 Fatty Acid. http://en.wikipedia.org/wiki/Fatty_acids. Accessed: April 9, 2013.

21 Månsson LH: Fatty acids in bovine milk fat. Food Nutr Res DOI: 10.3402/fnr.v52i0.1821.

22 Aggett PJ, Haschke F, Heine W, Hernell O, Koletzko B, Launiala K, Rey J, Rubino A, Schöch, Senterre J, et al: Comment on the content and composition of lipids in infant formulas. ESPGAN Committee on Nutrition. Acta Paediatr Scand 1991;80:887–896.

23 Klein CJ: Nutrient requirements for preterm infant formulas. J Nutr 2002;132:1395S–1577S.

24 Carnielli VP, Luijendijk IH, Van Goudoever JB, Sulkers EJ, Boerlage AA, Degenhart HJ, Sauer PJ: Structural position and amount of palmitic acid in infant formulas: effects on fat, fatty acid, and mineral balance. J Pediatr Gastroenterol Nutr 1996;23: 553–560.

25 Lindquist S, Hernell O: Lipid digestion and absorption in early life: an update. Curr Opin Clin Nutr Metab Care 2010;13:314–320.

26 Schanler RJ: Special methods in feeding the preterm infant; in Tsang RC, Nichols BL (eds): Nutrition During Infancy. Philadelphia, Hanley & Belfus, 1988, p 314.
27 Whyte RK, Campbell D, Stanhope R, Bayley HS, Sinclair JC: Energy balance in low birth weight infants fed formula of high or low medium-chain triglyceride content. J Pediatr 1986;108:964–971.
28 Wu PY, Edmond J, Auestad N, Rambathla S, Benson J, Picone T: Medium-chain triglycerides in infant formulas and their relation to plasma ketone body concentrations. Pediatr Res 1986;20:338–341.
29 Wirth FH Jr, Numerof B, Pleban P, Neylan MJ: Effect of lactose on mineral absorption in preterm infants. J Pediatr 1990;117:283–287.
30 Schulzke SM, Patole SK, Simmer K: Long-chain polyunsaturated fatty acid supplementation in preterm infants. Cochrane Database Syst Rev 2011;CD000375.
31 Coppa GV, Zampini L, Galeazzi T, Gabrielli O: Prebiotics in human milk: a review. Dig Liver Dis 2006;38:S291–S294.
32 Ziegler EE, Fomon SJ: Lactose enhances mineral absorption in infancy. J Pediatr Gastroenterol Nutr 1983;2:288–294.
33 Auricchio S, Rubino A, Muerset G: Intestinal glycosidase activities in the human embryo, fetus, and newborn. Pediatrics 1965;35:944–954.
34 Kien CL: Digestion, absorption, and fermentation of carbohydrates in the newborn. Clin Perinatol 1996;23:211–228.
35 Szylit O, Maurage C, Gasqui P, Popot F, Favre A, Gold F, Borderon JC: Fecal short-chain fatty acids predict digestive disorders in premature infants. JPEN J Parenter Enteral Nutr 1998;22:136–141.
36 Erasmus HD, Ludwig-Auser HM, Paterson PG, Sun D, Sankaran K: Enhanced weight gain in preterm infants receiving lactase-treated feeds: a randomized, double-blind, controlled trial. J Pediatr 2002;141:532–537.
37 Griffin MP, Hansen JW: Can the elimination of lactose from formula improve feeding tolerance in premature infants? J Pediatr 1999;135:587–592.
38 Committee on Nutrition of the Preterm Infant, European Society of Paediatric Gastroenterology and Nutrition: Nutrition and feeding of preterm infants. Acta Paediatr Scand Suppl 1987;336:1–14.
39 Atkinson S, Tsang RC: Calcium and phosphorus; in Tsang RC, Uay R, Koletzko B, Zlotkin SH (eds): Nutrition of the Preterm Infant: Scientific Basis and Practice, ed 2. Cincinnati, Digital Educational Publishing, 2005, pp 245–275.
40 Rigo J, Pieltain C, Salle B, Senterre J: Enteral calcium, phosphate and vitamin D requirements and bone mineralization in preterm infants. Acta Paediatr 2007;96:969–974.
41 Widdowson EM, McCance RA, Spray CM: The chemical composition of the human body. Clin Sci 1951;10:113–115.
42 Abrams SA: Calcium absorption in infants and small children: methods of determination and recent findings. Nutrients 2010;2:474–480.
43 Hicks PD, Rogers SP, Hawthorne KM, Chen Z, Abrams SA: Calcium absorption in very low birth weight infants with and without bronchopulmonary dysplasia. J Pediatr 2011;158:885–890.
44 Lapillonne AA, Glorieux FH, Salle BL, Braillon PM, Chambon M, Rigo J, Putet G, Senterre J: Mineral balance and whole body bone mineral content in very low-birth-weight infants. Acta Paediatr Suppl 1994;405:117–122.
45 Rigo J, De Curtis M: Disorders of calcium, phosphorus and magnesium metabolism; in Martin RJ, Fanaroff AA (eds): Neonatal-Perinatal Medicine: Diseases of the Fetus and the Infant. Philadelphia, Mosby Elsevier, 2006, pp 1491–1522.
46 Koo WW, Tsang RC: Mineral requirements of low-birth-weight infants. J Am Coll Nutr 1991;10:474–486.
47 Dauncey MJ, Shaw JC, Urman J: The absorption and retention of magnesium, zinc, and copper by low birth weight infants fed pasteurized human breast milk. Pediatr Res 1977;11:1033–1039.
48 Roy RN, Chance GW, Radde IC, Hill DE, Willis DM, Sheepers J: Late hyponatremia in very low birth-weight infants (less than 1.3 kilograms). Pediatr Res 1976;10:526–531.
49 Lozoff B, Beard J, Connor J, Barbara F, Georgieff M, Schallert T: Long-lasting neural and behavioral effects of iron deficiency in infancy. Nutr Rev 2006;64:S34–S43.
50 Hirano K, Morinobu T, Kim H, Hiroi M, Ban R, Ogawa S, Ogihara H, Tamai H, Ogihara T: Blood transfusion increases radical promoting non-transferrin bound iron in preterm infants. Arch Dis Child Fetal Neonatal Ed 2001;84:F188–F193.
51 Obladen M, Sachsenweger M, Stahnke M: Blood sampling in very low birth weight infants receiving different levels of intensive care. Eur J Pediatr 1988;147:399–404.
52 McDonald MC, Abrams SA, Schanler RJ: Iron absorption and red blood cell incorporation in premature infants fed an iron-fortified infant formula. Pediatr Res 1998;44:507–511.
53 Dauncey MJ, Davies CG, Shaw JC, Urman J: The effect of iron supplements and blood transfusion on iron absorption by low birthweight infants fed pasteurized human breast milk. Pediatr Res 1978;12:899–904.
54 Moody GJ, Schanler RJ, Abrams SA: Utilization of supplemental iron by premature infants fed fortified human milk. Acta Paediatr 1999;88:763–767.

55 Siimes MA, Vuori E, Kuitunen P: Breast milk iron – a declining concentration during the course of lactation. Acta Paediatr Scand 1979;68:29–31.
56 Committee on Nutrition, American Academy of Pediatrics: Nutritional needs of the preterm infant; in Kleinman RE (ed): Pediatric Nutrition Handbook, ed 6. Elk Grove Village, American Academy of Pediatrics, 2009, p 79.
57 Widdowson EM, Southgate DA, Hey E: Fetal growth and body composition; in Lindblad BS (ed): Perinatal Nutrition. New York, Academic Press, 1988, pp 3–14.
58 Hambidge M: Human zinc deficiency. J Nutr 2000; 130:1344S–1349S.
59 Ehrenkranz RA, Gettner PA, Nelli CM, Sherwonit EA, Williams JE, Ting BT, Janghorbani M: Zinc and copper nutritional studies in very low birth weight infants: comparison of stable isotopic extrinsic tag and chemical balance methods. Pediatr Res 1989;26: 298–307.
60 Sievers E, Oldigs HD, Dörner K, Schaub J: Longitudinal zinc balances in breast-fed and formula-fed infants. Acta Paediatr 1992;81:1–6.
61 Rao R, Georgieff MD: Microminerals; in Tsang RC, Uauy R, Koletzko B, Zlotkin SH (eds): Nutrition of the Preterm Infant: Scientific Basis and Practical Guidelines, ed 2. Cincinnati, Digital Educational Publishing, Inc., 2005, pp 277–310.
62 Tyrala EE: Zinc and copper balances in preterm infants. Pediatrics 1986;77:513–517.
63 Bannister WH: From haemocuprein to copper-zinc superoxide dismutase: a history on the fiftieth anniversary of the discovery of haemocuprein and the twentieth anniversary of the discovery of superoxide dismutase. Free Radic Res Commun 1988;5:35–42.
64 Casey CE, Neville MC, Hambidge KM: Studies in human lactation: secretion of zinc, copper, and manganese in human milk. Am J Clin Nutr 1989;49:773–785.
65 Schanler RJ, Shulman RJ, Lau C: Feeding strategies for premature infants: beneficial outcomes of feeding fortified human milk versus preterm formula. Pediatrics 1999;103:1150–1157.
66 Darlow BA, Austin NC: Selenium supplementation to prevent short-term morbidity in preterm neonates. Cochrane Database Syst Rev 2003;CD003312.
67 Makhoul IR, Sammour RN, Diamond E, Shohat I, Tamir A, Shamir R: Selenium concentrations in maternal and umbilical cord blood at 24–42 weeks of gestation: basis for optimization of selenium supplementation to premature infants. Clin Nutr 2004;23: 373–381.
68 Friel JK, Andrews WL, Long DR, Herzberg G, Levy R: Thiamine, riboflavin, folate, and vitamin B12 status of infants with low birth Weights receiving enteral nutrition. J Pediatr Gastroenterol Nutr 1996;22: 289–295.
69 Friel JK, Bessie JC, Belkhode SL, Edgecombe C, Steele-Rodway M, Downton G, Kwa PG, Aziz K: Thiamine, riboflavin, pyridoxine, and vitamin C status in premature infants receiving parenteral and enteral nutrition. J Pediatr Gastroenterol Nutr 2001;33: 64–69.
70 Körner RW, Müller C, Roth B, Vierzig A: Thiamin status of premature infants assessed by measurement of thiamin diphosphate in whole blood. Br J Nutr 2012;1:1–8.
71 Massey V: The chemical and biological versatility of riboflavin. Biochem Soc Trans 2000;28:283–296.
72 Moore MC, Greene HL, Phillips B, Franck L, Shulman RJ, Murrell JE, Ament ME: Evaluation of a pediatric multiple vitamin preparation for total parenteral nutrition in infants and children. I. Blood levels of water-soluble vitamins. Pediatrics 1986;77:530–538.
73 Raiten D, Talbot JM, Waters JH: Assessment of nutrient requirements for infant formulas. J Nutr Suppl 1998;128:2059S–2294S.
74 Porcelli PJ, Adcock EW, DelPaggio D, Swift LL, Greene HL: Plasma and urine riboflavin and pyridoxine concentrations in enterally fed very-low-birth-weight neonates. J Pediatr Gastroenterol Nutr 1996;23:141–146.
75 Borschel M: Vitamin B6 in infancy: requirements and current practices; in Raiten J (ed): Vitamin B6 in Pregnancy, Lactation and Infancy. Boca Raton, CRC Press, 1995, pp 109–124.
76 Vaz Pinto A, Torras V, Sandoval JF, Dillman E, Mateos CR, Córdova MS: Folic acid and vitamin B12 determination in fetal liver. Am J Clin Nutr 1975;28: 1085–1086.
77 Picciano MF: Water soluble vitamins in human milk; in Jensen R (ed): Handbook of Milk Composition. New York, Academic Press, 1995, pp 189–194.
78 Haiden N, Klebermass K, Cardona F, Schwindt J, Berger A, Kohlhauser-Vollmuth C, Jilma B, Pollak A: A randomized, controlled trial of the effects of adding vitamin B12 and folate to erythropoietin for the treatment of anemia of prematurity. Pediatrics 2006;118:180–188.
79 Koletzko B, Baker S, Cleghorn G, Neto UF, Gopalan S, Hernell O, Hock QS, Jirapinyo P, Lonnerdal B, Pencharz P, Pzyrembel H, Ramirez-Mayans J, Shamir R, Turck D, Yamashiro Y, Zong-Yi D: Global standard for the composition of infant formula: recommendations of an ESPGHAN coordinated international expert group. J Pediatr Gastroenterol Nutr 2005;41:584–599.
80 Darlow BA, Buss H, McGill F, Fletcher L, Graham P, Winterbourn CC: Vitamin C supplementation in very preterm infants: a randomised controlled trial. Arch Dis Child Fetal Neonatal Ed 2005;90:F117–F122.

81 Mactier H, Weaver LT: Vitamin A and preterm infants: what we know, what we don't know, and what we need to know. Arch Dis Child Fetal Neonatal Ed 2005;90:F103–F108.
82 Gross S, Melhorn DK: Vitamin E, red cell lipids and red cell stability in prematurity. Ann N Y Acad Sci 1972;203:141–162.
83 Greer FR: Vitamin metabolism and requirements in the micropremie. Clin Perinatol 2000;27:95–118.
84 Rossi R, Albrecht O, Pollmann H, Jorch G, Harms E: Effect of a reduced vitamin K supplementation on prothrombin time in prematures and high-risk neonates. Acta Paediatr 1996;85:747–749.
85 Gray TK, Lowe W, Lester GE: Vitamin D and pregnancy: the maternal-fetal metabolism of vitamin D. Endocr Rev 1981;2:264–274.
86 Agarwal R, Virmani D, Jaipal ML, Gupta S, Gupta N, Sankar MJ, Bhatia S, Agarwal A, Devgan V, Deorari A, Paul VK; Investigators of LBW Micronutrient Study Group, Departments of Pediatrics and Endocrinology: Vitamin D status of low birth weight infants in Delhi: a comparative study. J Trop Pediatr 2012;58:446–450.
87 Dawodu A, Nath R: High prevalence of moderately severe vitamin D deficiency in preterm infants. Pediatr Int 2011;53:207–210.
88 Taylor SN, Wagner CL, Fanning D, Quinones L, Hollis BW: Vitamin D status as related to race and feeding type in preterm infants. Breastfeed Med 2006;1:156–163.
89 Council on Environmental Health and Section on Dermatology: Ultraviolet radiation: a hazard to children and adolescents. Pediatrics 2011;127:588–597.
90 Hillman LS, Haddad JG: Perinatal vitamin D metabolism. II. Serial 25-hydroxyvitamin D concentrations in sera of term and premature infants. J Pediatr 1975;86:928–935.
91 Delmas PD, Glorieux FH, Delvin EE, Salle BL, Melki I: Perinatal serum bone Gla-protein and vitamin D metabolites in preterm and fullterm neonates. J Clin Endocrinol Metab 1987;65:588–591.
92 McCarthy RA, McKenna MJ, Oyefeso O, Uduma O, Murray BF, Brady JJ, Kilbane MT, Murphy JF, Twomey A, Donnell CP, Murphy NP, Molloy EJ: Vitamin D nutritional status in preterm infants and response to supplementation. Br J Nutr 2012;27:1–8.
93 Nako Y, Tomomasa T, Morikawa A: Risk of hypervitaminosis D from prolonged feeding of high vitamin D premature infant formula. Pediatr Int 2004; 46:439–443.
94 Pittard WB 3rd, Geddes KM, Hulsey TC, Hollis BW: How much vitamin D for neonates? Am J Dis Child 1991;145:1147–1149.
95 Markestad T, Aksnes L, Finne PH, Aarskog D: Vitamin D nutritional status of premature infants supplemented with 500 IU vitamin D2 per day. Acta Paediatr Scand 1983;72:517–520.
96 Hillman LS, Hollis B, Salmons S, Martin L, Slatopolsky E, McAlister W, Haddad J: Absorption, dosage, and effect on mineral homeostasis of 25-hydroxycholecalciferol in premature infants: comparison with 400 and 800 IU vitamin D2 supplementation. J Pediatr 1985;106:981–989.
97 Steichen JJ, Tsang RC, Greer FR, Ho M, Hug G: Elevated serum 1,25 dihydroxyvitamin D concentrations in rickets of very low-birth-weight infants. J Pediatr 1981;99:293–298.
98 Koo WW, Sherman R, Succop P, Ho M, Buckley D, Tsang RC: Serum vitamin D metabolites in very low birth weight infants with and without rickets and fractures. J Pediatr 1989;114:1017–1022.
99 Ravid A, Koren R, Rotem C, Amir Y, Reisner S, Novogrodsky A, Liberman UA: Mononuclear cells from human neonates are partially resistant to the action of 1,25-dihydroxyvitamin D. J Clin Endocrinol Metab 1988;67:755–759.
100 Evans JR, Allen AC, Stinson DA, Hamilton DC, St. John Brown B, Vincer MJ, Raad MA, Gundberg CM, Cole DE: Effect of high-dose vitamin D supplementation on radiographically detectable bone disease of very low birth weight infants. J Pediatr 1989;115:779–786.
101 Koo WW, Krug-Wispe S, Neylan M, Succop P, Oestreich AE, Tsang RC: Effect of three levels of vitamin D intake in preterm infants receiving high mineral-containing milk. J Pediatr Gastroenterol Nutr 1995;21:182–189.
102 Backström MC, Mäki R, Kuusela AL, Sievänen H, Koivisto AM, Ikonen RS, Kouri T, Mäki M: Randomised controlled trial of vitamin D supplementation on bone density and biochemical indices in preterm infants. Arch Dis Child Fetal Neonatal Ed 1999;80:F161–F166.
103 Backström MC, Mäki R, Kuusela AL, Sievänen H, Koivisto AM, Koskinen M, Ikonen RS, Mäki M: The long-term effect of early mineral, vitamin D, and breast milk intake on bone mineral status in 9- to 11-year-old children born prematurely. J Pediatr Gastroenterol Nutr 1999;29:575–582.
104 Kislal FM, Dilmen U: Effect of different doses of vitamin D on osteocalcin and deoxypyridinoline in preterm infants. Pediatr Int 2008;50:204–207.
105 Aine L, Backström MC, Mäki R, Kuusela AL, Koivisto AM, Ikonen RS, Mäki M: Enamel defects in primary and permanent teeth of children born prematurely. J Oral Pathol Med 2000;29:403–409.
106 Wagner CL, Greer FR; American Academy of Pediatrics Section on Breastfeeding; American Academy of Pediatrics Committee on Nutrition: Prevention of rickets and vitamin D deficiency in infants, children, and adolescents. Pediatrics 2008; 122:1142–1152.

107 Nucleotide. http://en.wikipedia.org/wiki/Nucleotide. Accessed: April 28, 2013.
108 Yu VY: The role of dietary nucleotides in neonatal and infant nutrition. Singapore Med J 1998;39:145–150.
109 Carver JD: Dietary nucleotides: effects on the immune and gastrointestinal systems. Acta Paediatr 1999;430:83–88.
110 Aggett P, Leach JL, Rueda R, MacLean WC Jr: Innovation in infant formula development: a reassessment of ribonucleotides in 2002. Nutrition 2003;19:375–384.
111 Choline. http://en.wikipedia.org/wiki/Choline. Accessed: April 28, 2013.
112 Rohlfs EM, Garner SC, Mar M-H, Zeisel SH: Glycerophosphocholine and phosphocholine are the major choline metabolites in rat milk. J Nutr 1993;123:1762–1768.
113 Inositol. http://en.wikipedia.org/wiki/Inositol. Accessed: April 28, 2013.
114 Pereira GR, Baker L, Egler J, Corcoran L, Chiavacci R: Serum myoinositol concentrations in premature infants fed human milk, formula for infants, and parenteral nutrition. Am J Clin Nutr 1990;S1:S89–S93.
115 Lewin LM, Melmed S, Passwell JH, Yannai Y, Brish M, Orda S, Boichis H, Bank H: Myoinositol in human neonates: serum concentrations and renal handling. Pediatr Res 1978;12:3–6.
116 Greene DA, Lattimer SA, Sima AAF: Sorbitol, phosphoinositides and sodium-potassium-ATPase in the pathogenesis of diabetic complications. N Engl J Med 1987;316:599–606.
117 Hailman M, Jarvenpaa AL, Pahjavuori M: Double-blind randomized trial of myoinositol supplementation in respiratory distress syndrome. Pediatr Res 1986;20:41.
118 Howlett A, Ohlsson A: Inositol for respiratory distress syndrome in preterm infants. Cochrane Database Syst Rev 2003;CD000366.
119 DiBiasie A: Evidence-based review of retinopathy of prematurity prevention in VLBW and ELBW infants. Neonatal Netw 2006;25:393–403.
120 Mugambi MN, Musekiwa A, Lombard M, Young T, Blaauw R: Probiotics, prebiotics infant formula use in preterm or low birth weight infants: a systematic review. Nutr J 2012;11:58.
121 Chauhan M, Henderson GM, McGuire W: Enteral feeding for very low birth weight infants: reducing the risk of necrotising enterocolitis. Arch Dis Child Fetal Neonatal Ed 2008;93:F162–F166.
122 Probiotics. http://en.wikipedia.org/wiki/Probiotic. Accessed: April 28, 2013.
123 Deshpande G, Rao S, Patole S: Probiotics for prevention of necrotising enterocolitis in preterm neonates with very low birthweight: a systematic review of randomised controlled trials. Lancet 2007;369:1614–1620.
124 Prebiotics. http://en.wikipedia.org/wiki/Prebiotic_(nutrition). Accessed: April 28, 2013.

Francis B. Mimouni, MD
Tel Aviv Medical Center, Dana Dwek Children's Hospital
6, Weizman Street
IL–64239 Tel Aviv (Israel)
E-Mail fbmimouni@gmail.com

Mimouni FB, van den Anker JN (eds): Neonatal Pharmacology and Nutrition Update.
Pediatr Adolesc Med. Basel, Karger, 2015, vol 18, pp 108–123 (DOI: 10.1159/000365035)

Neonatal Pharmacotherapy: Legal and Regulatory Issues

Ralph Bax · Paolo Tomasi

Paediatric Medicines, Product Development Scientific Support Department, European Medicines Agency, Canary Wharf, London, UK

Abstract

Off-label and unlicensed use of medicines is high in the paediatric population and specifically high in neonatal/paediatric intensive settings with up to 90% of cases. This is associated with higher incidence and severity of adverse drug reactions and can be addressed by including all paediatric age groups including neonates into clinical trials to ensure safety and efficacy of the medicine together with a formulation appropriate for the neonate. Legislation has been introduced in the US and the EU to request this development. A number of supporting scientific guidelines, network and further legal/regulatory initiatives are ongoing and have led to an increase of studies planned for neonates. However, even more efforts specifically for the most vulnerable and heterogeneous population of preterm infants is needed.

Introduction

Until a few decades ago, the sales and advertising of medicinal products were not regulated, meaning products could be sold even in the absence of minimal data on their safety, let alone efficacy. This led to a number of well-publicised public health disasters, many of which affected children and neonates.

For example, in 1937, an elixir of sulphanilamide (a sulphamide antibiotic product) was developed for use in children [1]. Diethylene glycol was chosen as a solvent, as it is odourless, sweet, and syrupy. Unfortunately, diethylene glycol is also highly toxic; it may cause vomiting, diarrhoea, cramps, dehydration, metabolic acidosis, renal and hepatic failure, seizures, and death. More than one hundred people died in the USA, many of them children, and this event was a major factor in the regulation of medicines in the USA (the passing, in 1938, of the Federal Food, Drug, and Cosmetic Act).

In 1956, newborns receiving sulphisoxazole were found to have a higher incidence of kernicterus, which only occurs in neonates or very young children. Until 1956, it was not known that sulphisoxazole displaces bilirubin from plasma proteins, thus increasing the free fraction of bilirubin in the plasma and enhancing the passage of bilirubin into the brain.

Other examples of unexpected neonatal toxicities include chloramphenicol (1959, grey baby syndrome) [2], benzyl alcohol (1982, neonatal gasping syndrome) [3], and vitamin E (1985, neonatal sepsis and necrotising enterocolitis) [4].

It is important to note that most of the regulatory principles for the authorisation of medicines in Europe were developed and applied in the wake of the thalidomide disaster, where more than 10,000 children were born with deformities such as phocomelia after maternal thalidomide use by the time of its initial withdrawal in 1961 [5].

Off-Label or Unlicensed Use of Medicines

Off-label use can be defined as the practice of prescribing pharmaceuticals for an unapproved indication or for an unapproved age group, unapproved dose, or unapproved form of administration [6]. In other words, an otherwise authorised medicinal product is considered to be used off-label when its use in a given patient group (e.g. neonates) and for a certain condition/disease occurs in the absence of specific authorisation granted by a regulatory body, such as the Food and Drug Administration (FDA) in the USA, National Competent Authorities in each of the EU member states or the European Medicines Agency (EMA); an unlicensed or unauthorised product has no authorisation at all in a given jurisdiction.

Because of the regulatory definition of off-label use, it follows that certain use of a medicinal product may be off-label in a jurisdiction (for example, a country in the European Union (EU)) but not in another (e.g. another country in the EU, China or Australia), depending on the degree of harmonisation of the different marketing authorisations in those jurisdictions.

Furthermore, in many cases, it may not be immediately clear to the practicing clinician if a medicinal product is in fact authorised for use in neonates for a given indication: the therapeutic indication reported in the product information (e.g. the Summary of Product Characteristics or the 'label') may not mention any age subgroup, and the posology may not help, for example, if expressed in dose per weight units. However, accurate consultation of the available information in the 'label' or on the websites of the regulatory authorities will usually reveal if studies in neonates have been performed that support the clinical use of the medicine in this subgroup.

Off-Label Use and Need for Clinical Trials in Neonates

Before the 1970s, children and pregnant women were routinely excluded from clinical trials of medicinal products, and 'protection' of children, 'a vulnerable population', and their 'inability to provide informed consent' were most often mentioned as justification. However, one wonders whether the practical difficulties of enrolling and studying children, and particularly neonates, may have contributed to this position.

Therefore, the vast majority of the use of medicinal products in neonates occurs off-label, particularly in intensive care and surgical settings [7–10].

Of course, off-label use does not necessarily imply arbitrary use without any support from clinical data; in fact, neonatology is one of the fastest developing areas and is an example of a success story in medicine. In this respect, while the prescribing of drugs in neonates can be off-label in 25–90% of cases [8–10], in a percentage of these cases, there was some scientific support in the literature for their use [11].

Nevertheless, unauthorised and off-label use of medicinal products are associated with a greater incidence and seriousness of adverse events [12, 13] and occur in a situation where the efficacy is also undemonstrated, which renders any toxicity unacceptable. In addition, underreporting of adverse events occurring with off-label use of medicines in children has also been described [3]. In light of the lack of controlled studies, the prescription of unauthorised or off-label drugs on the basis of some evidence, experience and extrapolation from adults or of the presumed efficacy in other paediatric age groups could be seen on one hand as the physician's duty – or on the other hand, if no change of this practice is encouraged, as a 'medical hazardous attitude' resulting in the physician being responsible for harming neonates [14].

In fact, off-label prescription may be considered, in certain jurisdictions and under certain circumstances (such as the absence of any published scientific support of the use), as an unauthorised clinical trial with potential legal consequences.

The pharmacological disasters mentioned above make it clear that safe and rational prescribing of drugs to children requires controlled studies of drugs in children, particularly in neonates [15], a proposal that many considered anathema just one generation ago. These studies should be followed by appropriate regulatory approval.

Need for clinical trials in neonates

A vulnerable population that is often treated with multiple medicines at the same time (up to 60 [13])

Just like children are not small adults, neonates are not small children; therefore, extrapolation of efficacy or safety from older children is very often inappropriate.

Neonates are the paediatric population for which less data on the correct use of medicines are available [16].

Gradual maturation of metabolic and detoxifying pathways during the first months of life causes different sensitivities and responses to active substances and excipients.

Ethical and scientific arguments in favour of protecting children through clinical trials, not from them

Higher incidence and severity of adverse drug reactions in the off-label use of medicinal products [12, 13]

Efficacy cannot be assumed when prescribing medicines that have not been tested in the appropriate population.

Inclusion of a child in a clinical trial is likely to be associated with a better outcome [16–18].

Failure to conduct clinical trials in children is unethical, as it forces physicians to do uncontrolled experiments almost every time they prescribe a medicine to a child.

Current Legal and Regulatory Status of the Prescription of Medicines to Neonates

In the Western world, the regulatory and prescription status of medicines in neonates is not in principle different from that in adults: in the USA and in the EU, a medicine can be marketed for a specific therapeutic indication (or for prevention or diagnosis) only if its benefit-risk profile has been deemed to be satisfactory by a regulatory body (often called an 'agency'). In the USA, this role is almost exclusively covered by the FDA, whereas in the EU, a decentralised system of national agencies, coordinated by the EMA and the European Commission, exerts the same role.

Evaluation of the benefit-risk profile is based on three main pillars: the quality of the product (the manufacturing of the active substance[s] and of the final product on the shelves, its physico-chemical and stability characteristics, etc.), its safety, and its efficacy towards the specific indication(s).

Currently, the assessment of the benefit-risk for each indication is done for separate populations, so in principle, a medicine in a given indication may be authorised, for example, for adults only, for adults and children, or for neonates only (exceptionally, e.g. surfactant therapy for respiratory distress syndrome in newborn premature infants), and not for the whole population from birth to extreme old age. However, this has not been the case in all jurisdictions in the past, so in many instances, authorisations were granted without specification of an age group but almost always in the absence of any data in neonates (or older children) and very often without an explicit posology for neonates (or older children).

As already mentioned, it may not be easy to define in precise legal terms which use of a medicinal product in neonates (or children) can be considered 'on-label' and which is considered off-label. The question is, however, of important practical relevance because, in some jurisdictions, off-label use may be forbidden, subjected to specific clauses (e.g. need for written informed consent), or not reimbursed by third-party payers.

Because legislation can differ widely in different countries/jurisdictions, practitioners should make themselves familiar with the regulatory and legal framework in the region where they operate. It is beyond the scope of this chapter to describe in detail the existing differences, even in a single, relatively uniform area such as the EU (28 jurisdictions at the moment of writing); however, two examples of different ways of addressing the issue of off-label prescription in neonates will be provided (Italy and France, see below).

From a scientific point of view, it can be accepted that off-label use in neonates occurs whenever a health professional uses a medicinal product that is not explicitly authorised in this age group, and at the same time, the product information (label) contains no information on the posology or safety and efficacy in neonates for that indication.

Medical treatment of neonates occurs almost exclusively in a hospital setting and not at home or in the community, as is often the case for older children. In many countries/jurisdictions, this usually translates into more freedom to prescribe and use medicinal products off-label, for example if national legislation or the payer's rules prevent reimbursement of the product when prescribed off-label in the pharmacy.

Making Neonatal Pharmacotherapy 'Legal': Two Different Approaches

Off-label use is not limited to neonates, of course, and in some countries/jurisdictions, attempts have been made to regulate and to a degree allow the use of selected products under specific circumstances. Two examples of this are the recently enacted or modified legislations in France and Italy.

France

A new legislative framework with the aim to reduce and regulate off-label drug use for adults as well as for children was implemented in France (Law number 2011–2012, December 29, 2011) together with a related decree for 'Temporary Recommendations for Use' (TRUs; Decree number 2012–743, May 9, 2012) [20].

The legislation has provided 'a regulatory process for temporarily supervising the prescribing of drugs for indications for which they are not yet licensed' [20]. A TRU can be granted for a maximum of 3 years to open an observational window to assess benefit and risk and to collect scientific information. However, the manufacturer is expected to apply for authorisation of the indication at the end of the 3-year period after having acquired sufficient data. A TRU is issued a single time for any given drug, and this decision may grant reimbursement for the designated indication. The French Medicines Agency will authorise a TRU (only) if there are no other appropriate medications available.

The legislation may potentially encourage the development of potential new uses for marketed drugs and the monitoring of benefit-risk ratios for new indications or new patient groups, including neonates. The potential disadvantage is that once a new use has been temporarily authorised, it may then be difficult to stop physicians from prescribing the drug for that indication, even if a new market authorisation is not eventually granted.

At the moment, it is too early to assess any impacts of this new legislation, particularly for the neonatal population.

Italy

Traditionally, hospital physicians in Italy had been allowed to prescribe medicines off-label to inpatients, while office-based general practitioners and community paediatricians were not. However, recent legislative changes meant that physicians prescribing off-label were liable to reimburse the cost of the products to the National Health Service out of their own pockets, even when this was done for inpatients. As in neonatology and neonatal and paediatric anaesthesia, off-label use is the rule rather than the exception. The financial implications for neonatologists and paediatric anaesthesiologists were substantial, and these two groups asked the Italian Medicines Agency to find a solution.

Even though this new legislation was subsequently allowed to expire, the Italian Medicines Agency decided to use an existing law (648/1996) that allowed reimbursement of medicinal products for off-label use under certain conditions. The law had been developed mainly to allow cancer patients to receive expensive new products free of charge when the process for authorisation of a new indication was ongoing or when the product, while authorised in the EU, was not yet marketed in Italy.

Separate groups of paediatric specialists therefore conducted an analysis of the existing literature for the neonatal and paediatric use of approximately 20 medicinal products (guidelines, scientific publications, use in other countries, etc.), which were then listed for reimbursement in new off-label indications by state law in August 2012 [21].

It is important to note that this 'approval' is only applicable to reimbursement; the indication remained technically off-label, which had several important consequences, among which two must be mentioned:

(1) the lack of specific indication means that the use was still off-label, thus requiring (in Italy) explicit informed consent (a particularly problematic issue in neonatology and neonatal/paediatric anaesthesia); and

(2) as the new indication is not included in the Summary of Product Characteristics, it could not be easily extended to other countries in the EU by means of existing regulatory pathways (such as the Mutual Recognition Procedure [22]).

Legislation to Facilitate the Development of Medicines for Neonates

The fact that the use of medicines in neonates occurs very often off-label and often without any substantial data on the dose, safety or efficacy of the use is now acknowledged by scientists and legislators in the EU, the USA and, more generally, in the whole world.

However, the development of medicines for children in general, and even more so for neonates, is in most circumstances not economically rewarding for the pharmaceutical companies; in addition, it is fraught with other practical difficulties (recruiting issues, commitment of healthcare professionals, vulnerable population with assent/consent difficulties, etc.).

For these reasons, both the EU and the USA have adopted legislation to increase the number of approved indications of medicines in children and neonates.

The USA opened the way with two different acts, the Best Pharmaceutical for Children Act (BPCA) and the Pediatric Research Equity Act (PREA), which have recently become permanent (2012). More recently, in the EU, the Paediatric Regulation entered into force in 2007.

Both approaches provide a system of obligations and incentives for pharmaceutical companies. In the EU, for example, paediatric development is now in principle mandatory for every new medicinal product, unless the pharmaceutical company obtains an exemption (called a waiver), for example, because the product is not considered safe for or advantageous to children (or because the indication does not apply to children, say for the treatment of Alzheimer's disease).

Dedicated regulatory paediatric frameworks, as in the USA and the EU, have not been implemented in other regions, especially not in high-income regions. For example, discussions in Australia are ongoing [23].

More details on the incentives, obligations and other dispositions in the USA and the EU are reported below.

US Legislation

Because children and particularly neonates have been underrepresented in clinical trials for the proof of efficacy and safety of drugs, regulatory and legal initiatives were first successfully launched in the USA by the National Institutes of Health (NIH) and the FDA in the 1990s, which resulted in the Pediatric Pharmacology Research Units Network, the FDA Modernization Act (1997), the BPCA (2002), the PREA (2003), and the FDA Amendments Act (2007), which reauthorised the BPCA and PREA [24]. In 2012, provisions to the BPCA and PREA were made permanent by the Food and Drug Administration Safety and Innovation Act [25].

In summary, the BPCA provides an optional financial incentive to conduct trials in children, at the request of the FDA, in the form of an accelerated approval process and an additional 6 months of market exclusivity.

The PREA on the other hand allows the FDA to require (impose) paediatric studies for the same indication(s) for which authorisation is sought in adults, without providing a reward, unless a waiver for studies is granted by the FDA.

Following these legislative initiatives, an increase in paediatric studies has been observed, and 467 paediatric labelling changes have been recorded in the FDA's 'New Pediatric Labeling Information Database' (as of February 2013) [26].

The situation for neonates, however, is less encouraging, with 30 products including neonates in the studies and 25 products with neonatal information in the labelling (as of October 2012 [26]). The situation for preterm neonates is even worse; they have only been involved in one study. This is also reflected in the clinicaltrials.gov database, with 22.2% of all trials including children (out of 142,303 recorded trials, as of March 2013) and only 1.5% including neonates [27].

In 2012, the Food and Drug Administration Safety and Innovation Act identified the need to include the neonatal population and imposed additional obligations on the need to justify any exclusion of neonates from developments done in the framework of the BPCA reward and requiring neonatology expertise in the Office of Pediatric Therapeutics at the FDA [28, 29].

European Union Legislation

A European Paediatric Regulation was introduced in 2006 and gradually entered into force in 2007 and 2008 [30] to address the need for better paediatric development of medicinal products. A Regulation is the strongest type of EU law, as it is immediately applicable in all EU member states. The provisions of the regulation offer similar incentives as the US legislation because an extension of the patent protection for 6 months for products with a completed agreed paediatric development can be requested; the requirements and obligations, however, are slightly different, as the EU legislation also applies to orphan drugs and to existing (already authorised) products.

For the initial authorisation of new products in the EU (regardless of the approval route: centralised or non-centralised), companies will have to obtain approval from the EMA for the studies to be done with neonates or children well in advance of their application for marketing authorisation in adults, i.e. usually before safety and efficacy studies are started in adults. This is compulsory for all products, unless when an exemption (waiver) is granted by the EMA.

Studies in neonates and children need not necessarily be done at the same time as in adults, as deferrals can be granted when appropriate. In practice, this happens in more than 80% of cases.

Pharmaceutical companies need to discuss all paediatric age groups, particularly those including neonates and describe the development of neonatal age-appropriate formulations as well as the required specific, non-clinical and clinical development (if any) for all paediatric age subsets in their applications to obtain approval for the studies in a Paediatric Investigation Plan (PIP).

The Paediatric Regulation includes further measures to support paediatric drug development by providing information and transparency, and by stimulating research. Scientific advice for the development of paediatric medicines is offered free of charge and can be sought at any time during the development [31]. For transparency, all paediatric clinical trial studies performed in the EU and worldwide (if part of a PIP) will be registered on the EU database [32], which can be accessed via a dedicated EU clinical trials register website [33].

An EMA survey on the use of medicines in children in Europe confirmed that newborn and preterm newborn neonates are the age group with the highest reported unauthorised/off-label use [16].

An analysis of data gathered between January 2007 and December 2011 [34] showed that neonatal drug development has been specifically mentioned to agree a PIP in approximately in one of four applications. This seems to be a low number; however, it might reflect the fact that the majority of conditions and indications targeted by the applicants do not exist in neonates, whereas development in adolescents, for example, is only rarely waived. The Paediatric Committee at the EMA has encouraged the inclusion of neonates into the development plans, resulting in almost doubling the percentage of PIPs including neonatal studies compared to the initial proposal of pharmaceutical companies (from 15 to 28% in January to October 2008 [35] and from 24 to 32% in March to December 2011 [34]).

For the off-patent medicine initiative, over half of all 15 projects funded by the European Commission under the 7th Framework Programme until January 2012 specifically concerned the development of medicines for neonates [36].

Development of Medicines for and Clinical Trials in Neonates: Legislative, Regulatory and Ethical Framework

Every year, an estimated 4 million infants die in the neonatal period, and the proportion of neonatal mortality is increasing (38% of all child deaths in 2000), with 99% of neonatal deaths arising in low- to middle-income countries [37]. In these areas, efforts are first needed to build capacity as a basis for a legislative and regulatory framework for the regulatory oversight and assessment of paediatric trials [23].

In 2007, the World Health Assembly resolution 'Better Medicines for Children' (WHA60.20) recognised the need for research in and development of medicines for children, including the need to undertake activities such as improving research, regulation, access and rational use [38]. Therefore, the WHO launched a campaign in 2007 'Make medicines child size' and published the third model list of essential medicines for children in 2011, which also contains medicines for use in neonates and a section for 'specific medicines for neonatal care' [39]. Based on this, a model formulary for children was developed [40]. In 2008, the Paediatric Medicines Regulators' Network, comprised of representatives of national regulatory authorities including the FDA and EMA, was set up by the WHO to develop regulatory capacity for the development of paediatric medicines, e.g. by providing a platform for discussing paediatric drug development and specific training including neonatal issues [41].

Paediatric drug development is a complex undertaking, and this is especially true for neonatal drug development due to the heterogeneous population including the group of preterm infants. This group in itself is very heterogeneous, has the highest amount of developmental physiological changes occurring in a short time frame, has a high variability of pharmacological parameters and presents challenging practical and ethical issues for performing clinical trials. Thus, the neonatal population is in a way the 'orphan' of the 'therapeutic orphans' [42], being the most vulnerable population, with a history of being neglected by all stakeholders, including investigators, industry and regulatory agencies. Therefore, a systematic approach is of utmost importance, particularly for this population [43], and regulators have taken the approach not only to provide and enforce legislation but also to offer interdisciplinary platforms to advance and encourage systematic drug development in neonates.

Scientific Guidelines

Especially in areas with scarce experience such as neonatal drug development, the provision of requirements and incentives, which in general have shown to be successful, is not sufficient to encourage ethical and high-quality research in these areas. Therefore, regulatory initiatives include further measures, of which the ones important for neonatal drug development are highlighted in the following section.

Pharmaceutical companies are expected to follow the regulatory guidelines when developing medicinal products unless appropriate justification is provided. While the principles contained in the regulatory guidelines are not mandatory (from either a legal or regulatory standpoint), it is considered that non-observance should be occasional and justified.

In the US, the Newborn Drug Development Initiative was created by the National Institute of Child Health and Human Development and the FDA in 2003 [44]. The outcomes for different areas, e.g. neurology, cardiology, drug prioritisation and ethics, were published [45]. Similar efforts were provided by EMA with workshops on neonatology and expert meetings on neonatal and paediatric sepsis [46]. Concept papers on the impact of brain [47], lung and heart [48], liver [49] and renal [50] immaturity on the development of medicinal products were developed, and a general guideline on the investigation of medicinal products in term and preterm neonates was published [51]. Specific guidance for studies in neonates is also increasingly being included in general regulatory scientific guidelines, such as for persistent pulmonary hypertension of the newborn [52].

Neonatal (Age-Appropriate) Pharmaceutical Forms and Formulations

As widely recognised, the development of an age-appropriate formulation for neonates is specifically challenging [53]. In this respect, critical issues with significant potential impact on safety and toxicity include, for example, acceptable excipients for this vulnerable age group, administration via naso-gastric tube for liquid formulations, and amount of volume to be administered intravenously, especially for preterm neonates.

To support this development, regulatory authorities have published specific guidance; recently, for example, a 'Guideline on pharmaceutical development of medicines for paediatric use' [54].

Non-Clinical Development

The inclusion of the youngest paediatric age groups into clinical trials is expected to lead to a higher number of juvenile animal studies. This indeed has been confirmed in an analysis of 97 PIPs between November 2008 and May 2011 [55], and scientific guidance has been published by regulatory agencies both in the USA [56] and EU [57].

Clinical Development

Clinical trials in neonates are especially challenging regarding methodological, operational and ethical issues.

Often an age-staggered approach is used, which has the advantage of first gathering essential safety and efficacy in older age groups before including neonates in trials. On the other hand, this might delay the development of medicines for this age group or even render later trials impossible, as off-label use might have developed in the mean time and because parents and investigators might not be willing to include newborns in trials.

Apart from the scientific guidelines giving advice for specific conditions, as discussed above, there is further general guidance, which is particularly important for conducting studies in neonates. For example, there is guidance requiring the minimisation of blood-sampling volume that states that blood loss should not exceed 3% of the total blood volume or 1% of the blood volume at any single time [58]. Regulators increasingly encourage modelling and simulation methods, including physiologically based pharmacokinetic (PK) modelling, population PK approaches with sparse sampling, pharmacokinetic/pharmacodynamic (PK/PD) modelling and adaptive designs, and Bayesian approaches. This is also reflected in a number of regulatory guidance documents [59]. Furthermore discussions regarding the possibility of avoiding unnecessary trials in neonates in cases where, for example, efficacy data could be extrapolated from older age groups, are ongoing [60, 61].

Ethical Aspects

Ethical aspects are tightly interwoven with legal, regulatory, methodological and scientific concerns about pharmaceutical development and treatment in neonates and children. Many regulatory and legal provisions on the administration of medicines to neonates and children are based on ethical concerns.

Ethical concerns are particularly relevant in neonatal clinical trials due to many factors, including the impossibility of obtaining assent from the child, their high vulnerability, the time constraints that are often faced in an intensive care/neonatal setting, and the physical and mental status of the parents (who need to express consent). Fetal research poses still additional, specific ethical problems [62].

To further complicate the issue, ethical concepts may vary importantly across time and/or space; what is considered ethical now in Western Europe may be not acceptable in China, India or the USA, or even within Western Europe in the past (or in the future). As a practical example, in a few European jurisdictions, clinical studies that do not have the possibility to grant a direct benefit to the participants, such as some single-dose pharmacokinetics-only studies, are considered unethical and are therefore not legally or regulatorily allowed in neonates or children.

The ethical aspects of clinical trials in neonates and children are discussed in several documents, from the Declaration of Helsinki [63] to the guideline E11 of the International Conference on Harmonization [64]. More recently, a document on 'Ethical considerations for clinical trials on medicinal products conducted with the paediatric population' has been published on the European Commission's website by a European 'ad-hoc' group, and its conclusions are expected to be endorsed in PIPs agreed on by the EMA [58].

The ethical aspects of paediatric studies, with emphasis also on neonatal studies, have been discussed in recent workshops organised by the NIH in 2009 and by the EMA in 2011 [65, 66].

However, the discussion on the ethical aspects of routine medicinal product use in neonates is less developed. In practice, clinicians often find themselves in an uncomfortable position, and the frequent need to use products off-label is an ethical conundrum associated with potential medico-legal and civil liability risks, whether the final decision is to administer the product or not [14].

As discussed above, the only long-term solution consists of obtaining appropriate and reliable data on the safety and efficacy of medicines in neonates (and indeed in all paediatric age groups) with the appropriately authorised indications after evaluation by regulatory bodies. In neonates, a specific type of clinical trial, the so-called 'opportunistic studies', may be employed to at least collect information on safety and dosing, if not efficacy, in situations where the use of a comparator would be deemed unethical or inappropriate [67]. In an opportunistic study, a child receives an off-patent or understudied therapeutic agent as part of standard of care and, after informed consent, investigators collect PK samples at the time of routine laboratory draws or using scavenged samples. Low-volume sampling and population-PK (sparse sampling) methods would be preferred in these studies.

Conclusion

Neonatologists, paediatricians, paediatric anaesthesiologists and all healthcare providers involved in the care of neonates need to be thoroughly familiar with the legal and regulatory framework of the jurisdiction in which they operate. Substantial differences in regulation exist among countries/states that might have a substantial impact, financial or legal, on practitioners.

Published evidence consistently shows that administration of medicinal products in neonates occurs very often in the absence of approval for their use for the specific condition and that, in a substantial percentage of these cases, no scientific evidence supports the use of the medicines in this vulnerable population.

This is because, in general, medicinal products are not studied sufficiently in neonates, for a number of historical and market reasons.

Legislative approaches in the US and EU have addressed this, and preliminary data show that these paediatric regulatory frameworks have increased the number of paediatric trials and of authorised neonatal/paediatric indications for new or existing medicines. However, the situation in the most vulnerable population, term and preterm neonates, can still be improved.

All stakeholders need to be involved and engaged, i.e. industry must engage in neonatal trials, investigators and physicians must include neonates in clinical trials, and regulators must encourage and request these trials. Specifically, more efforts have to be made, even for the most vulnerable population, the preterm newborns.

Disclaimer

The views presented in this chapter are those of the authors and should not be understood or quoted as being made on behalf of the EMA and/or its scientific committees.

References

1 Ballentine C: Taste of raspberries, taste of death: the 1937 elixir sulfanilamide incident. FDA Consumer Magazine 1991. http://www.fda.gov/AboutFDA/WhatWeDo/History/ProductRegulation/SulfanilamideDisaster/default.htm (accessed March 2013).

2 Sutherland JM: Fatal cardiovascular collapse of infants receiving large amounts of chloramphenicol. AMA J Dis Child 1959;97:761–767.

3 Gershanik J, Boecler B, Ensley H, McCloskey S, George W: The gasping syndrome and benzyl alcohol poisoning. N Engl J Med 1982;307:1384–1388.

4 Johnson L, Bowen FW Jr, Abbasi S, Herrmann N, Weston M, Sacks L, Porat R, Stahl G, Peckham G, Delivoria-Papadopoulos M, Quinn G, Schaffer D: Relationship of prolonged pharmacologic serum levels of vitamin E to incidence of sepsis and necrotizing enterocolitis in infants with birth weight 1,500 g or less. Pediatrics 1985;75:619–638.

5 Emanuel M, Rawlins M, Duff G, Breckenridge A: Thalidomide and its sequelae. Lancet 2012;380:781–783.

6 Stafford RS: Regulating off-label drug use–rethinking the role of the FDA. N Engl J Med 2008;358:1427–1429.

7 Conroy S, McIntyre J, Choonara I: Unlicensed and off label drug use in neonates. Arch Dis Child Fetal Neonatal Ed 1999;80:F142–F144.

8 Dell'Aera M, Gasbarro AR, Padovano M, Laforgia N, Capodiferro D, Solarino B, Quaranta R, Dell'Erba AS: Unlicensed and off-label use of medicines at a neonatology clinic in Italy. Pharm World Sci 2007;29:361–367.

9 Lindell-Osuagwu L, Korhonen MJ, Saano S, Helin-Tanninen M, Naaranlahti T, Kokki H: Off-label and unlicensed drug prescribing in three paediatric wards in Finland and review of the international literature. J Clin Pharm Ther 2009;34:277–287.

10 Kimland E, Nydert P, Odlind V, Böttiger Y, Lindemalm S: Paediatric drug use with focus on off-label prescriptions at Swedish hospitals – a nationwide study. Acta Paediatr 2012;101:772–778.

11 Doherty DR, Pascuet E, Ni A, Stewart P, Splinter W, Vaillancourt R: Off-label drug use in pediatric anesthesia and intensive care according to official and pediatric reference formularies. Can J Anaesth 2010;57:1078–1088.

12 European Medicines Agency: Evidence of harm from off-label or unlicensed medicines in children. http://www.ema.europa.eu/docs/en_GB/document_library/Other/2009/10/WC500004021.pdf (accessed March 2013).
13 Turner S, Nunn AJ, Fielding K, Choonara I: Adverse drug reactions to unlicensed and off-label drugs on paediatric wards: a prospective study. Acta Paediatr 1999;88:965–968.
14 D'Aloja E, Paribello F, Demontis R, Müller M: Off-label drugs prescription in neonatology: a physician's duty or a medical hazardous attitude? J Matern Fetal Neonatal Med 2011;24(suppl 1):99–100.
15 Giacoia GP, Taylor-Zapata P, Zajicek A: Drug studies in newborns: a therapeutic imperative. Clin Perinatol 2012;39:11–23.
16 European Medicines Agency: Report on the survey of all paediatric uses of medicinal products in Europe. http://www.ema.europa.eu/docs/en_GB/document_library/Report/2011/01/WC500101006.pdf (accessed March 2013).
17 Meadows AT, Kramer S, Hopson R, Lustbader E, Jarrett P, Evans AE: Survival in childhood acute lymphocytic leukemia: effect of protocol and place of treatment. Cancer Invest 1983;1:49–55.
18 Stiller CA, Draper GJ: Treatment centre size, entry to trials, and survival in acute lymphoblastic leukaemia. Arch Dis Child 1989;64:657–661.
19 Janni W, Kiechle M, Sommer H, Rack B, Gauger K, Heinrigs M, Steinfeld D, Augustin D, Simon W, Harbeck N, Friese K; ADEBAR Study Group: Study participation improves treatment strategies and individual patient care in participating centers. Anticancer Res 2006;26:3661–3667.
20 Emmerich J, Dumarcet N, Lorence A: France's new framework for regulating off-label drug use. N Engl J Med 2012;367:1279–1281.
21 Agenzia Italiana del Farmaco: Normativa di riferimento – Sperimentazione clinica; Farmaci off label (L.648/96). http://www.agenziafarmaco.gov.it/it/content/normativa-di-riferimento-sperimentazione-clinica (accessed September 2014).
22 European Commission: The mutual recognition procedure. http://ec.europa.eu/health/authorisation-procedures-mutual-recognition_en.htm (accessed March 2013).
23 Hoppu K, Anabwani G, Garcia-Bournissen F, Gazarian M, Kearns GL, Nakamura H, Peterson RG, Ranganathan SS, de Wildt SN: The status of paediatric medicines initiatives around the world – what has happened and what has not? Eur J Clin Pharmacol 2012;68:1–10.
24 FDA: Memorandum: establishment of the Pediatric Review Committee (PeRC). http://www.fda.gov/downloads/Drugs/DevelopmentApprovalProcess/DevelopmentResources/UCM049871.pdf (accessed March 2013).
25 OpenCongress: H.R. 4274 (112th) – BPCA and PREA Reauthorization Act of 2012. http://www.opencongress.org/bill/hr4274-112/show (accessed September 2014).
26 FDA: New pediatric labelling information database. http://www.accessdata.fda.gov/scripts/sda/sdNavigation.cfm?sd=labelingdatabase (accessed March 2013).
27 ClinicalTrials.gov. http://www.clinicaltrials.gov (accessed March 2013).
28 FDA: 2013 Meeting materials, Pediatric Advisory Committee to the Food and Drug Administration: March 15, 2013 meeting of the Neonatology Subcommittee of the Pediatric Advisory Committee. http://www.fda.gov/AdvisoryCommittees/CommitteesMeetingMaterials/PediatricAdvisoryCommittee/ucm341096.htm (accessed March 2013).
29 FDA: Neonatology Subcommittee of the Pediatric Advisory Committee meeting. http://www.fda.gov/downloads/AdvisoryCommittees/CommitteesMeetingMaterials/PediatricAdvisoryCommittee/UCM342926.pdf (accessed March 2013).
30 Regulation (EC) No 1901/2006 of the European Parliament and of the Council of 12 December 2006 on medicinal products for paediatric use and amending Regulation (EEC) No 1768/92, Directive 2001/20/EC, Directive 2001/83/EC and Regulation (EC) No 726/2004. http://ec.europa.eu/health/files/eudralex/vol-1/reg_2006_1901/reg_2006_1901_en.pdf (accessed March 2013).
31 European Medicines Agency: Scientific advice and protocol assistance. http://www.ema.europa.eu/ema/index.jsp?curl=pages/regulation/general/general_content_000049.jsp&mid=WC0b01ac05800229b9 (accessed March 2013).
32 EudraCT. https://eudract.ema.europa.eu/ (accessed in March 2013).
33 EU clinical trials register. https://www.clinicaltrialsregister.eu/ (accessed March 2013).
34 European Medicines Agency: 5-year report to the European Commission: general report on the experience acquired as a result of the application of the Paediatric Regulation. http://ec.europa.eu/health/files/paediatrics/2012-09_pediatric_report-annex1-2_en.pdf (accessed March 2013).
35 Olski TM, Lampus SF, Gjerarducci G, Saint Raymond A: Three years of paediatric regulation in the European Union. Eur J Clin Pharmacol 2011;67:245–252.
36 European Commission: FP7 funded projects for off-patent medicines for children. http://cordis.europa.eu/search/result_en?q='off-patent'%20AND%20'children'%20AND%20contenttype='project'%20AND%20programme/code='FP7-HEALTH'%20AND%20sicCode/code='MED'%20AND%20language='en' (accessed September 2014).

37 Lawn JE, Cousens S, Yupan J; Lancet Neonatal Survival Steering Team: 4 million neonatal deaths: When? Where? Why? Lancet 2005;365:891–900.
38 Sixtieth World Health Assembly: Resolution WHA60.20: Better medicines for children. http://apps.who.int/gb/ebwha/pdf_files/WHA60/A60_R20-en.pdf (accessed March 2013).
39 World Health Organization: WHO model list of essential medicines for children, 4th list, April 2013. http://apps.who.int/iris/bitstream/10665/93143/1/EMLc_4_eng.pdf?ua=1 (accessed September 2014).
40 World Health Organization: WHO model formulary for children. http://apps.who.int/medicinedocs/documents/s17151e/s17151e.pdf (accessed September 2014).
41 World Health Organization: Paediatric medicines Regulators' Network PmRN. http://www.who.int/childmedicines/paediatric_regulators/en/ (accessed March 2013).
42 Shirkey H: Therapeutic orphans. J Pediatr 1968;72: 119–120.
43 Turner MA: Neonatal drug development. Early Hum Dev 2011;87:763–768.
44 Giacoia GP, Mattison MD: Newborns and drug studies: The NICHD/FDA Newborn Drug Development Initiative. Clin Ther 2005;27:796–813.
45 Giacoia GP, Mattison DR: Selected proceedings of the NICHD/FDA newborn drug development initiative: Part II. Clin Ther 2006;928:1337–1341.
46 European Medicines Agency: Pediatric medicines: workshops. http://www.ema.europa.eu/ema/index.jsp?curl=pages/regulation/general/general_content_000416.jsp&mid=WC0b01ac0580118a19 (accessed March 2013).
47 European Medicines Agency: Concept paper on the impact of brain immaturity when investigating medicinal products intended for neonatal use. http://www.ema.europa.eu/docs/en_GB/document_library/Scientific_guideline/2009/09/WC500003800.pdf (accessed March 2013).
48 European Medicines Agency: Concept paper on the impact of lung and heart immaturity when investigating medicinal products intended for neonatal use. http://www.ema.europa.eu/docs/en_GB/document_library/Scientific_guideline/2009/09/WC500003802.pdf (accessed March 2013).
49 European Medicines Agency: Concept paper on the impact of liver immaturity when investigating medicinal products intended for neonatal use. http://www.ema.europa.eu/docs/en_GB/document_library/Scientific_guideline/2009/09/WC500003803.pdf (accessed March 2013).
50 European Medicines Agency: Concept paper on the impact of renal immaturity when investigating medicinal products intended for neonatal use. http://www.ema.europa.eu/docs/en_GB/document_library/Scientific_guideline/2009/09/WC500003807.pdf (accessed March 2013).
51 European Medicines Agency: Guideline on the investigation of medicinal products in the term and preterm neonate. http://www.ema.europa.eu/docs/en_GB/document_library/Scientific_guideline/2009/09/WC500003750.pdf (accessed March 2013).
52 European Medicines Agency: Paediatric addendum to CHMP guideline on the clinical investigations of medicinal products for the treatment of pulmonary arterial hypertension. http://www.ema.europa.eu/docs/en_GB/document_library/Scientific_guideline/2012/02/WC500122492.pdf (accessed March 2013).
53 Noel GJ, Van Den Anker JN, Lombardi D, Ward R: Improving drug formulations for neonates: making a big difference in our smallest patients. J Pediatr 2012;161:947–949.
54 European Medicines Agency: Guideline on pharmaceutical development of medicines for paediatric use: Draft. http://www.ema.europa.eu/docs/en_GB/document_library/Scientific_guideline/2013/01/WC500137023.pdf (accessed March 2013).
55 Carleer J, Karres J: Juvenile animal studies and paediatric drug development: a European regulator experience. Birth Defects Res B Dev Reprod Toxicol 2011;92:254–260.
56 FDA: Guidance for industry nonclinical safety evaluation of pediatric drug products. http://www.fda.gov/downloads/Drugs/GuidanceCompliance RegulatoryInformation/Guidances/ucm079247.pdf (accessed March 2013).
57 European Medicines Agency: Guideline on the need for non-clinical testing in juvenile animals of pharmaceuticals for paediatric indications. http://www.ema.europa.eu/docs/en_GB/document_library/Scientific_guideline/2009/09/WC500003305.pdf (accessed March 2013).
58 European Commmission: Ethical considerations for clinical trials on medicinal products conducted with the paediatric population. ftp://ftp.cordis.europa.eu/pub/fp7/docs/ethical-considerations-paediatrics_en.pdf (accessed March 2013).
59 Zisowsky J, Krause A, Dingemanse J: Drug development for pediatric populations: Regulatory aspects. Pharmaceutics 2010;2:364–388.
60 Dunne D, Rodriguez WJ, Murphy MD, Nhi Beasley B, Burckart GJ, Filie JD, Lewis LL, Sachs HC, Sheridan PH, Starke P, Yao LP: Extrapolation of adult data and other data in pediatric drug-development programs. Pediatrics 2011;128:e1242–e1249.

61 European Medicines Agency: Concept paper on extrapolation of efficacy and safety in medicine development: Draft. http://www.ema.europa.eu/docs/en_GB/document_library/Scientific_guideline/2012/06/WC500129285.pdf (accessed March 2013).
62 Russell BA, Cohen SN, Delaney-Black V: Ethics of drug research in pediatric populations; in Yaffe SJ, Aranda JV (eds): Neonatal and Pediatric Pharmacology, ed 4. Philadelphia, LWW, 2005, pp 99–100.
63 World Medical Association: World Medical Association Declaration of Helsinki: Ethical principles for medical research involving human subjects. http://www.wma.net/en/30publications/10policies/b3/17c.pdf (accessed March 2013).
64 European Medicines Agency: Note for guidance on clinical investigation of medicinal products in the paediatric population. http://www.emea.europa.eu/docs/en_GB/document_library/Scientific_guideline/2009/09/WC500002926.pdf (accessed March 2013).
65 NIH and FDA: Workshop on ethical and regulatory issues in global pediatric trials, September 20–22, 2009. http://bpca.nichd.nih.gov/collaborativeefforts/Documents/ethic_pediatric_09-20-2009.pdf (accessed March 2013).
66 European Medicines Agency: Ethical considerations for paediatric trials - how can ethics committees in the European Member States and the Paediatric Committee at the European Medicines Agency work together? http://www.ema.europa.eu/ema/index.jsp?curl=pages/news_and_events/events/2011/07/event_detail_000443.jsp&mid=WC0b01ac058004d5c3 (accessed March 2013).
67 Tibboel D: Trials with neonates: desirable scientific approaches, their ethical issues and potential solutions. http://www.ema.europa.eu/docs/en_GB/document_library/Presentation/2012/01/WC500120286.pdf (accessed March 2013).

Ralph Bax
Paediatric Medicines, Product Development Scientific Support Department
European Medicines Agency
30 Churchill Place
Canary Wharf, London E14 5EU (UK)
E-Mail ralph.bax@ema.europa.eu

Author Index

Subject Index